Running Your First
ULTRA

Customizable Training Plans
for Your First 50K to 100-Mile Race

Krissy Moehl

**A top female ultramarathon runner,
with more than 100 races and 55 wins to her name**

Photography by
Fredrik Marmsater

PAGE STREET
PUBLISHING CO.

First published in 2015 by

Page Street Publishing Co.

27 Congress Street, Suite 103

Salem, MA 01970

www.pagestreetpublishing.com

Distributed by Macmillan, sales in Canada by The Canadian Manda Group.

18   17   16   15   1   2   3   4   5

ISBN-13: 978-1-62414-142-3

ISBN-10: 1624141420

Library of Congress Control Number: 2015939748

Cover and book design by Page Street Publishing Co.

Printed and bound in China

Page Street is proud to be a member of 1% for the Planet. Members donate one percent of their sales to one or more of the over 1,500 environmental and sustainability charities across the globe who participate in this program.

Motivated by
Passion and Consistency,
life lessons learned from Ma & Pa Moehl
and reinforced with trail time.

Dedicated to
my treasured mentors
for their wisdom
and my coaching clients
for their newbie enthusiasm.

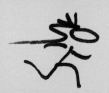

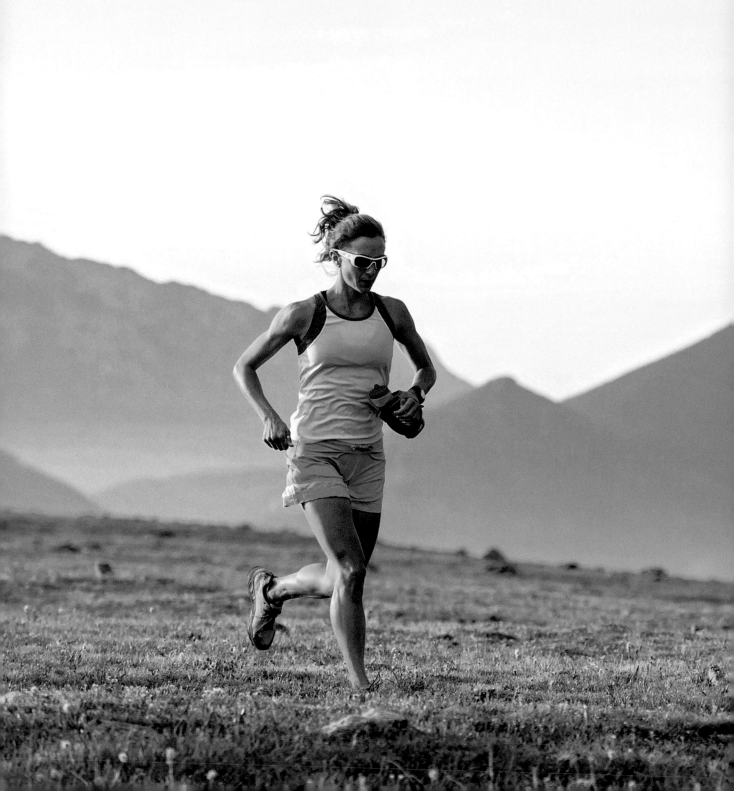

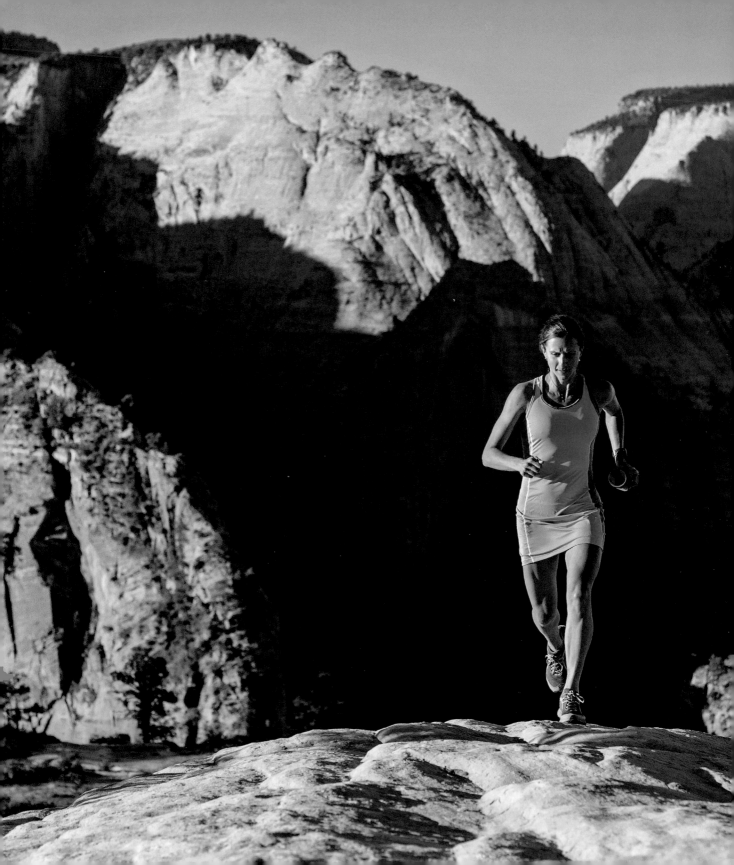

INTRODUCTION

Your first ultra has the potential to impact, change, mold and direct your life from this point forward. The amount of time you will put into your training and the perspective you can gain are not to be taken lightly. This is an exciting and challenging endeavor and one I hope to provide an obtainable, less daunting path to by sharing my experiences, both good and bad, to help you thrive in your first ultra.

In 1999, with pigtails and only 22 years of life experience, wonderment drew me into the sport of ultrarunning. Men ranging in age from young bucks to grizzly grays offered their hard-earned and learned lessons from their years on the trails. Absorbing their words of wisdom provided my start. Morphing the tips to work with my body made the sport enjoyable, possible and sustainable. Recognize the difference between a 48-year-old male and a 22-year-old female and understand the importance of tailoring your systems. Every body is different and it is important to figure out yours.

The growing ultra community is a gathering place for deeply motivated, outwardly laid back, welcoming souls. As you delve deeper you will find encouragement, amazing trail stories and challenges that will keep you coming back for more. Observing the community, you will find that ultrarunning is a lifestyle. Running and runners both will touch your life in an influential way. When kept in balance, the journeys and lessons will guide, sustain and contribute to your life. It is my goal to help you successfully integrate the wonder of this sport so that you identify as an Ultrarunner; to make it something that you are, not something that you do.

Writing this book is both a privilege and a joy. After 15 years, pigtails now braided, I feel I have grown up in this sport and in this community. I am thankful for its influence and consistency in my life. I feel lucky to be in a position to reflect on it all through the process of creating your training guide.

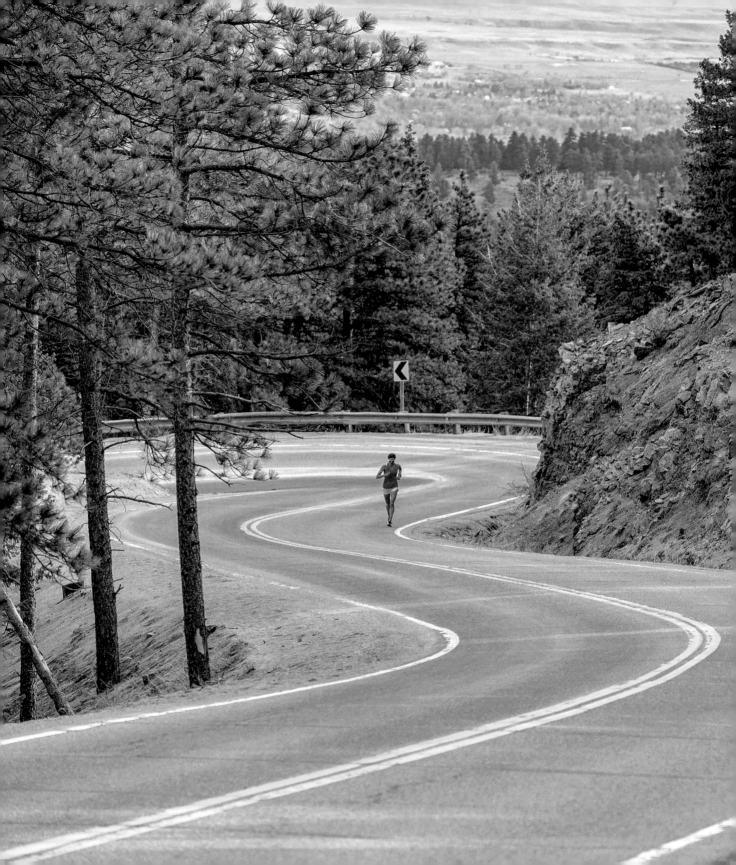

CHAPTER ONE

FINDING YOUR DISTANCE: ULTRAMARATHON Q&A

Taking on an ultra is an ambitious goal, whether it is your first or 50th. Ultrarunning takes commitment, motivation and that little something extra, to endure and enjoy your training and racing. If you are excited, driven and willing to put in the necessary time, you will surprise yourself with what you are able to accomplish. And, if you pay attention, you will learn a lot about training, your body and your mental fortitude through the process.

To start, it is important to me that you check in with your lifestyle. Answer the following questions. These are questions to keep in mind as you plan your first ultra. Tackling them up front will help you set appropriate expectations for you and those close to you.

Have you had a recent physical exam/fitness test?

Do you have enough time to train, recover and remain engaged with work and family?

Do you have access to trails/training grounds?

Will your finances support your goals?

Is this something you want to tackle alone or do you desire the support of your family and friends?

Will your chosen training plan work with your current day-to-day schedule or are there some life adjustments you need to consider? What are they?

What are areas of your life that can yield during high-mileage training weeks?

What is motivating you to run an ultra?

   a. I've run a marathon and I wonder what is next.

   b. My friends are running one and think I should too.

   c. I read a book about long-distance running, or talked to a long-distance runner, and it appeals to me.

   d. Personal reasons. Examples: Health, weight loss, relationship woes, addiction recovery, lifestyle change

   e. Other _____

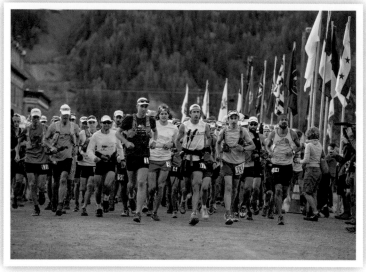

Hardrock 100 race start 2012

Next, check in with your current fitness. Do you have a reliable foundation from which to build toward your ultrarunning goals? Be honest. It is important to start your plan from the required base. Example: Do not jump into the 100-mile training plan if you are currently running 20-30 miles a week. (See notes at the start of each training plan.)

Finally, dial in your race goal. Perhaps you have already answered this question or maybe you are debating on where to start. Either way, answer the following questions honestly.

For each of the following questions, circle one answer (a-c) per question. Additionally, circle (d) if it applies.

Questions

1) Which distances have you raced in the last 5 months?

   a. 5k or 10k, half marathon, marathon

   b. A couple of marathons and/or 50ks

   c. 50 miler or 100 km

   d. Multiple 50ks and a couple 50 milers

2) How many days a week can you run? (Schedule-wise and physically)

   a. 3-4 days/week

   b. 4-5 days/week

   c. 5-6 days/week

   d. 6-7 days/week

3) What mileage range have you averaged for the past three months?

   a. 30-40 miles/week

   b. 40-50 miles/week

   c. 50-65 miles/week

   d. 65-80 miles/week

4) How much time do you have to train?

    a. 5-8 hours/week

    b. 8-10 hours/week

    c. 10-14 hours/week

    d. >14 hours/week

5) What type of terrain will you primarily train on? What is most accessible?

    a. Roads, dirt paths or single-track trails—relatively flat

    b. Answer (a) terrain during the week, single track, varied to hilly trails on weekends

    c. 40 percent time on answer (a) terrain, 60 percent on single-track trails (varied to hilly)

    d. 30 percent on answer (a) terrain, 60-70 percent on single-track trails (mountainous)

6) What does your life dynamic include? Family? Work? Social?

    a. I need to balance my training with work and family.

    b. Work OR family is demanding, but I have flexibility otherwise.

    c. My partner (and family) is (are) supportive. Work offers good flexibility.

    d. This is my main focus.

Tally your responses. If you have mostly (a) answers, turn to page 50 for a 24-week 50k training plan. If (b) answers dominate your scorecard, turn to page 78 and review your 24-week 50-mile or 100-km training plan. Finally, if you primarily answered (c), dig in to the 48-week 100-mile plan on page 105. Additionally, if you circled a minimum of two (d) answers, you can consider looking into more mountainous racecourses for any of the race distances.

I tend to train more effectively when I know the end goal. The next chapter will give you resources and tips on picking your first ultra race. Then you can plan your training to line up accordingly and start dreaming about toeing the line.

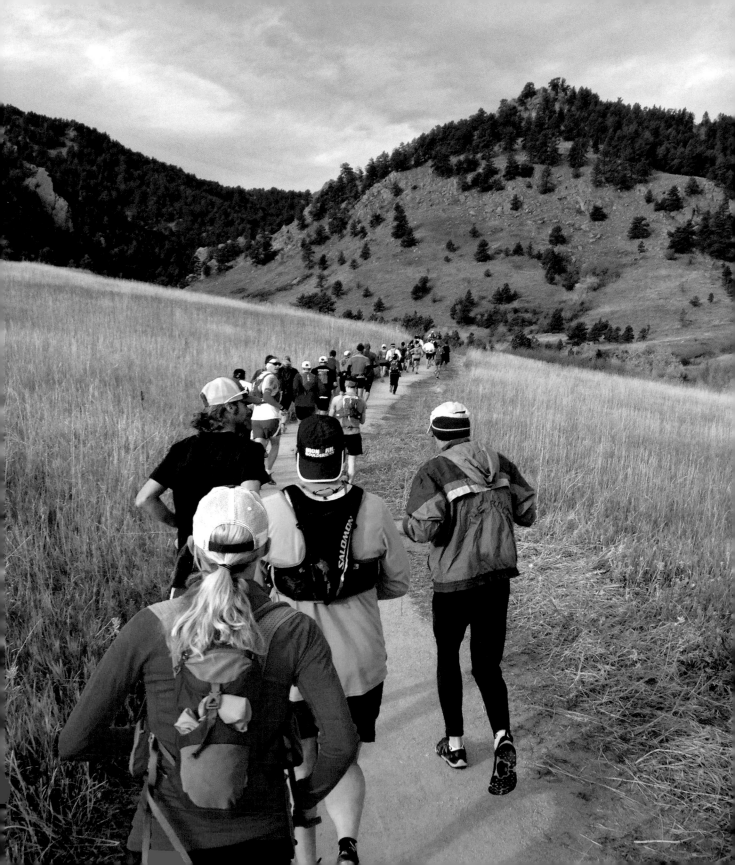

CHAPTER TWO

WHICH ONE WILL YOU RUN?

- ➜ *Distance (page 13)*
- ➜ *Location (page 13)*
- ➜ *Course Profile (page 13)*
- ➜ *Race History (page 14)*
- ➜ *Budgeting (page 14)*

It is important to remember that your first race will always hold a special place in your heart. Perhaps someone has already convinced you of the perfect first ultra. Or maybe you heard about a race years ago and it is finally time to step up and give it a try. It is exciting to look at race websites, course maps and elevation profiles as you dream about running your first ultra. When it comes time to choose your first race, there are a few key points to consider.

DISTANCE. The Ultramarathon Q&A (pg. 9) will guide you through a series of questions and help you reach a realistic first goal. If your initial dream when you picked up this book was to run 100 miles, but you are currently running 30 miles a week, use the training plans to guide you to that end goal. Build and improve your functional base, learn about your body and progress through the distances at a manageable rate. Ex: Train for your first 50-miler 3–5 months after your first 50k. Recover. And then build for your first 100-miler.

LOCATION. Do your ultra dreams include international or cross-country travel? Or does the race across town, starting at your local trailhead, spark your interest? While traveling to race is an amazing way to explore the world, and I have raced more destination races than local ones, I encourage you to simplify the details of your first race. Travel and expenses can add unnecessary pressure and stress to your experience. Choosing a local race, or one in a familiar location (Ex: visiting relatives or friends and tying in a race), ensures close-to-home comforts and supports your usual routine as the race approaches. Get your first ultra under your belt and then let the exploring begin! With the popularity of ultra and trail-running booming around the globe, there is no shortage of amazing race experiences to engage all the senses. The concerns (expense, travel, different foods, jetlag, etc.) are also what make the experience more involved, engaging and exciting.

COURSE PROFILE. Consider the terrain you have available on which to train when picking your race. To prepare for a challenging mountain run you will benefit by having access to long ascents, preferably steep and technical, in order to practice both climbing and descending. Likewise, training on gnarly mountains will not prepare you for smooth, flat, fast bike paths. For your first ultra, I suggest picking a race that mimics your training grounds. If you are determined to run a race that does not mimic your training grounds, then there are training methods using your local terrain to help prepare you for success. (See Chapter 14, What Is Next?, page 209, section Next Race.)

RACE HISTORY. Your first ultra race should be at a well-established event. First, look over the race website. Is there enough information to plan your weekend? Do you have running friends that can recommend the event? Look for race reports that describe the details of the event you are considering.

Choosing a reputable race increases your likelihood for success and enjoyment in your first ultra experience. Do the reports boast a top-notch event? Or do you read of complaints and mishaps? Is the same race director (or a similar race committee) in charge each year? Or is the event constantly changing hands? Is this a business that puts on multiple events each year? Do you want a classic, homegrown event, or a streamlined business model? And finally, look into how many years the event has been held; I think a minimum of two or three years gives a sufficient understanding. While new events are usually established with the best intentions, I do not recommend picking a first-time race for your first ultra. Much like you are figuring out the nuances, so too is a first-time race director. Better to let them work out the bugs and for you to choose an established event.

As the sport of ultrarunning grows and evolves, access to information about events is much more accessible. *Ultrarunning Magazine* used to be the only resource for race reports. Now the magazine would be a book each month if it published every submitted story. This wealth of information that overflows to many online resources and to multiple magazines is your homework. Your highest priorities should include a well-marked course, an accurately timed event and sufficiently stocked aid stations. Bonus touches include nice awards, a community inspired pre- and/or post-race event and sponsor presence.

CREATE A BUDGET. This is not completely necessary, but may be helpful. If you follow this step prior to starting your training, you can set realistic expectations (there may be a few more costs than you originally planned) and minimize financial stress. See page 225 for a race budget spreadsheet.

Final Thought: In March of 2000, I toed the line of my first ultra at the 8th annual Chuckanut 50km. The race initially started as an "If I can do it, you can do it" dare from a good buddy of mine and has resulted in my ongoing relationship to the event as the race director for 13 years (and still going!). My hope is that your first ultra will be filled with amazing memories and an ongoing connection.

➜ Scott Jurek makes the most of the limited oxygen in Colorado's San Juan Mountains.

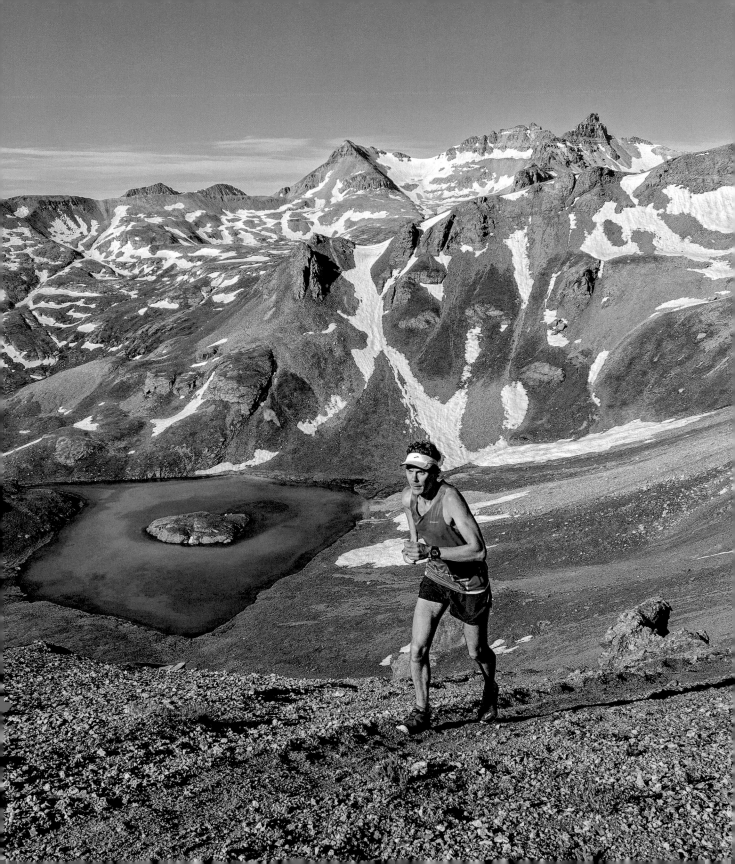

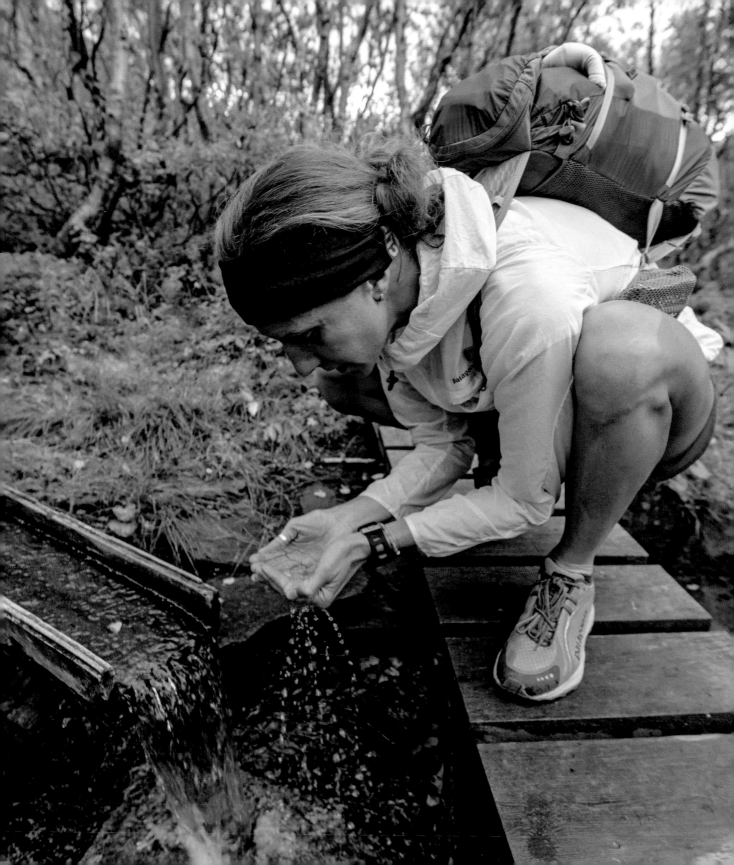

TRICKS OF THE TRADE

- -

There are lessons you have to learn the hard way by enduring the experience. Likewise, there are tips you can pickup from mentors to help you avoid unnecessary challenges. While the sometimes painful stories of how I came to learn the helpful tips in this section are entertaining, I hope by sharing them with you, your learning curve will be friendlier.

- -

THE ENVIRONMENT

The most important lesson to me is that as trail runners we are aware of our **environmental impact**. We have the ability to move through the land lightly. We carry less, we cover more ground and we are able to see the beauty of an area, in what might be a three-day hike for some, in a day. Typically we do not camp overnight or cook in the backcountry. As shared users in the variety of landscapes that our feet take us through, it is our job to ensure that the beauty remains intact. Try the approach of sneaking through and minimizing your toll on the land. Pick up garbage, do not break tree limbs or remove plants. Apply Leave No Trace™ principles wherever you are. Realize your impact on the environment and do what you can daily to minimize your footprint. This lesson is learned on the trail and applies to life. Beyond running, I hope these actions translate to your daily routine.

FOOT CARE

Our feet start the chain and are the most important link in successful training and racing. From the skin to the ligaments, it is important to give our feet detailed attention.

You will discover more about shoe and sock options in the Gear section (page 181) with specifics to form and gate. Here I address matching the contours of the shoe with the flex points of the foot. Finding the right **shoe** and sock combination that work well for your feet is the first step. Utilize the knowledge and help of the staff at a specialty run shop to steer you in the right direction. Lace up the shoe as you would to run and bend and flex your foot through heal strike and toe-off. Most specialty running stores will encourage you to run around the block. Take them up on that offer and see if you notice any hot spots. Double-check the inside (liner) of the shoe. Try it on barefoot and see if you notice any stitching or rough spots that have potential to rub your skin. If you say, "once they break in," then you should try a different shoe. There is a model that will work for you from the start.

The trick that works for me is a shoe that secures the heel and instep with a lacing system and inner structure to reduce excess (back-and-forth and side-to-side) movement in the shoe. A wider toe box allows my toes to splay out and not be forced to rub together. As you pick a shoe model, depend on the structure and fit to minimize your foot slipping around; do not choose a smaller size. It is important to allow space for the expansion of the foot for long-distance running. The secure heal and instep also offer structure as the miles increase. I believe this support helps reduce fatigue by limiting extra motion and stress caused when trying to maintain foot placement in a sloppy fitting shoe.

And as your stride, strength and feet change with time, it is always good to reassess. This is another good reason to maintain a relationship with your local running store.

As my feet toughened to the sport of ultrarunning, I tried a variety of methods to deal with the blisters that plagued my boney heels. In my first two years of ultraracing, I often silver lined my heels with duct tape to endure the horrible rubbing from the heel counter of my shoe. I do not recommend duct tape. Nearly every time I peeled it off, I reluctantly removed a few layers of skin leaving a pink, raw and sometimes bloody mess to deal with afterwards.

Good protection and traction underfoot go a long way to prevent stone bruising to the bottoms of the feet and to keep you upright on slabby rocks, in mud, snow or loose sand. A protection plate made of TPU or dense EVA foam through the midsole will help disperse the pressure of a sharp rock or unexpected root. The variety of rubber compounds and traction patterns adhere to the countless terrains. Accommodating your terrain is a great reason to have a quiver of shoes. My ideal situation with any piece of running gear is to not notice its presence because it is functioning perfectly with my body and the terrain.

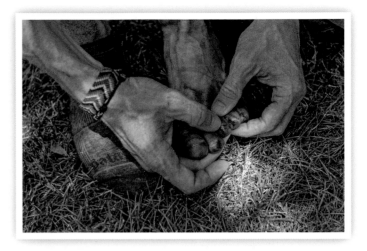

Fortunately, my feet continue to toughen over the years and miles. I have found sock (see Gear page 181) and shoe combinations that work and, most importantly, *I fix the little issues before they become big ones*. One trick I've added to my race day routine is to shake a tablespoon of 2 Toms Blistershield™ in each of my socks before putting them on. The directions call for a teaspoon; I prefer a substantial coating. I have found this keeps my feet dry and the skin less prone to the suppleness caused from sweat or water crossings. There are runners that swear by **skin lubes** and coat their feet in a variety of petroleum jelly-like products. I encourage you to find what works best for you by testing these options on your longer training runs.

The Important Extras for Feet

I am a firm believer in regular **pedicures** for everyone. The polish is a fun touch (and either coats nails preventing black toes, or at the very least hides them), but it is the soaking, scrubbing, de-callusing (more on this in a second), moisturizing and massaging aspects of a pedicure that are the most beneficial. You can do this for yourself or pay for the special treatment at a salon; the point is to take care of your feet.

Calluses are feedback relating where the most stresses are being placed on your feet and there are a variety of opinions on what to do about them. Some feel they are hard earned and protect our feet, while other runners are disgusted by excess, dead skin. I feel there is a happy medium and I tend toward the less-is-more end of the spectrum. A blister forming under an excessive callus is even more painful than a surface blister. And if there is structural pain to the foot associated with your calluses, consider adjustments to your running form and footwear.

To keep calluses to a minimum, but not completely removed, I find using the PedEgg™ (which is like a fine cheese grater for your feet) every two-three weeks works wonders (follow the instructions!). Finally, a personal secret to prevent black toes is to keep **toenails** clipped short and filed flat. I always clip, file and decoratively paint mine about one week out from a race or long run. Your feet do so much for you; it is wise to look out for them.

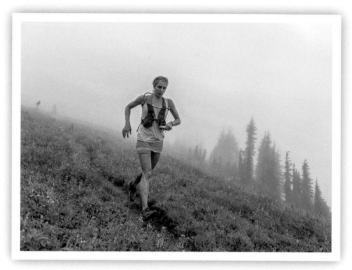

BODY CARE

The hardest lessons come when we first jump in, and they are the ones we remember the most.

There are numerous suggestions in this book's training plans to test out all of your gear before race day, especially on your long runs. Having your clothing realized can help you prevent the painful reality of **chafing**. Test out different fabrics in all weather conditions and for varying durations of time. Adjust your pack to prevent pressue points, make sure your hat fits but not too snug and that your sunglasses enhance rather than distort your vision. If chafing is unavoidable, look into Body Glide and other balms/lubricants. Reducing friction is your goal. Try compression (Gear chapter, page 184) on the run and to aid your recovery. You will find recommendations for apparel and layering (see Gear chapter, page 183 and Race Packing List, page 226) to prepare for varying weather conditions. Work with these suggestions, ask for recommendations from peers and find what works best for you.

Another skin-specific detail is **sunscreen**. Personally, growing up in the Pacific Northwest and not really knowing any better, sunscreen was not a priority. If I remembered or someone offered, I might smear some on my skin. Living in Colorado for the last three years, it is a part of my daily routine. I always wear it on my face, and I will put it on my neck, arms and legs if I am going to be in the sun for more than an hour. It was important to find a sunscreen that allows my skin to breathe and sweat. Sweat proof sunscreen has its benefits when you are sitting on a beach, but when you are hammering up a hill with the sun beating on your back, you need to sweat to keep your body cool. It is better to reapply than to block your skin's ability to breathe and cool. I am not married to a particular brand, but I am certain to test any before race day. I tend toward brands such as Rocket Pure Alba, Kin-e-sys, All Good Elemental Herbs, Sol and Kiss My Face.

My first ultra, the Chuckanut 50km in Fairhaven, Washington, was mid-March of 2000. Low, dark clouds unleashed sheets of rain while the wind blew sideways, ensuring that every square inch of clothing and skin was waterlogged. My Ma held her tongue while I waivered between shorts and tights only seconds before the race director sent us on our way. New shorts, an old university team issue sports bra, a thick tech fiber long sleeve shirt with a mock neck collar, a fleece vest and cotton gloves covered most of my body. This is not the kit I would wear today. Long story short, when I hobbled into the shower after the race, my depleted quads could not get me out of the streaming needles of hot water fast enough. My lower back, underarms and inner thighs were on fire! The wet clothing and movement from running wore off the top layer of skin. Let's just say I waited a day to scrub off the dirt.

As pedicures are important to your feet, so is **massage** to your body. As a trick of the trade, finding a licensed massage practitioner (LMP) who understands the runner's body, offers deep tissue work and is aware of the more easily aggravated "runner" points will make a significant difference in your treatment. Receiving a massage monthly at a minimum and twice a month in heavier training periods (weekly if you can afford it) will help you recover and keep your muscle fibers in proper alignment. I also suggest finding a LMP you like and stick with the same person. He/she will get to know you and your body and the bodywork will evolve to be more specific to your needs.

Sickness. If you catch a cold, stuffy head or cough, should you train through it? I find that if my symptoms are above my collarbone then I can typically train through, but I back off my workouts to about 80 percent of what I planned. It is important to maintain your hydration and core temperature, so drink, shower and change immediately after. Your hydration needs will increase to help flush the bug, so do not deplete yourself on your run. If symptoms are below the collarbone or the flu is involved, rest is best no matter where you are in your training plan. If you try to train through, chances are high that you will prolong and potentially worsen the illness. Your body will recover faster if you give it what it needs. Rest, hydrate, fuel and sleep. These are all things you are well-trained to do.

Now that we are comfortable with each other, and I've shared the easy to talk about tricks of the trade, it is time to bring up **bathroom talk**. As you talk about your longer training runs with people that do not spend hours in the woods, you will encounter lots of questions. Do not be surprised when people ask you, "How do you go the bathroom out there?" I will leave it up to you to figure out how you want to answer that. I'll offer some insight to my reality with a few short thoughts.

Remember my first ultra story? (See inset on the previous page) That painful shower afterwards? The part I emitted was that in my effort to save time and charge toward the win and new women's course record, I decided to pee myself rather than stop on the three-mile descent about nine miles from the finish. I know now, it was not worth the couple of seconds when I had minutes to spare! In my defense, my previous racing experience was college cross-country and a couple of seconds meant the difference of a team win.

My advice learned from this and other racing experiences is to always find an appropriate place to relieve yourself and do not soil your clothes in the process. An appropriate place requires awareness of your surroundings. Move away from all water sources. Bury your solids at least six inches deep. Do not be surprised when using outdoor facilities, compounded with longer running efforts, causes significant skin discomfort in your nether regions. Hopefully I do not need to explain in detail other than to suggest that Desitin may be your best friend and may save you in the long run. I learned this trick on the John Muir Trail and am forever grateful for my trail partner's advance wisdom so that we were well supplied. Do not leave TP anywhere; carry it out in the plastic baggie you brought it in. Be careful using natural TP alternatives: dead leaves, rocks or pinecones. Depending on your location, some plants, even when they are dead, have poisons that can cause mild to intense irritations. Harder objects like rocks and pinecones might abrade your skin. The best natural TP I've found is packable snow. Enough said.

Hydration and Nutrition

Considering the variety of environments you will train and race in, the adaptation your body makes through training and the inevitable caloric increase needed as your output rises, hydration and nutrition are the ever-changing and sometimes perplexing factors of running ultras. The human body is amazing and adapts by slowing metabolism to conserve energy for up to three hours of output without demanding replacement. To me, it is better to fuel and encourage my body rather than forcing it to adapt. This will benefit you as your distance and time on feet increases; your ability to fuel will be the difference in your performance. I believe good ultrarunners are good eaters. Do not forget, your daily (nutrition and hydration) requirements will also increase, in addition to what your training needs.

Your training environment, temperature, altitude and humidity levels will affect your **hydration needs**. Replacing adequate water and electrolytes is crucial. The ***Sweat Rate Test***[1] is a simple do-it-yourself trick that will keep you in tune with your body's fluid demands. First, weigh yourself dry and naked (you do not want the weight of wet hair). Then get dressed and go for a 1-hour run in your standard environment at a steady effort. Do not consume or expel any liquids other than sweat. (I advise you to use the bathroom first, and then weigh yourself.) When you return from your run, strip naked, dry yourself off and weigh yourself again. Every pound lost is equivalent to 16 oz of liquid that you need to replace per hour. If the color of your urine is darker than normal, not associated to supplements (example: vitamin B makes urine bright yellow), additional hydration is needed.

Hydration liquid replacement can be water or electrolyte drink. A combination of the two becomes more important as your running hours increase. Electrolytes can be replaced through formulated drinks, energy food products, pills and whole foods. Figuring out your specific electrolyte needs and replenishment options is a personal science. I encourage you to ask friends, read labels and studies, and test the variety of product options. Figure out what works for you while remaining open to the reality that your needs will change over time.

The next time you go on a run, repeat the Sweat Rate Test but drink the appropriate fluids and see if you can maintain your weight. If you put on weight, you are either drinking too much or it may be an indicator that your electrolytes are out of balance and you are retaining fluids, not peeing or sweating enough relative to your consumption. If you lose weight, remember it is water weight; you did not consume enough fluids. If you are running to lose weight, it will come with time, not after one run. Tuning in to your body and figuring out these needs are huge steps in understanding the finer details that will help you succeed in your ultra run.

Keep in mind your fluid quantities and product preferences will change as your fitness improves and as seasons change. Temperature, altitude, travel, humidity and what you eat prior to training (Ex: meals with higher sodium content) are all factors to be aware of in relation to your hydration needs. Use the Sweat Rate Test repeatedly to help learn your body and how it adapts. Over time, you will be able to make adjustments on intuition.

Fueling for an ultra run is tricky business as there is no umbrella formula that works for everyone and there are many factors at play. What you eat outside of running, any dietary restrictions, your body mass, gender and age all affect how you fuel on the run. Creating a relationship[2] with how food works in your body is key. This is formed by attentive eating and understanding how your body responds to the foods you eat. You may have aversions to dairy or meat. You may feel bloated when you eat certain foods. Figure out the nutrition that works for you by being aware of every aspect of your fuel—flavor, aroma, texture and most importantly how your body reacts each time you eat. Take notes and review them. After a short time, you will not have to think about it as much and you will be more familiar with fueling the demands of your training.

In studying my body at Seattle Performance Medicine in Seattle and reading runner books and magazines for years, I learned that most well-trained athletes most often burn between 600–1,000 calories/hour depending on their physical exertion. Our digestive system can process 200–400 calories per hour while in motion and upwards of 600 calories with training. A well-nourished athlete typically stores sufficient glycogen to fuel the energy demands of a run shorter than 90 minutes.[3] Training and fuel affect glycogen

1   American College of Sports Medicine; Sawka MN, et al. American College of Sports Medicine position stand. Exercise and fluid replacement. (2007) *Med Science Sports Exercise, 39,* 377-390.
2   Eisenstein, Charles (2003) *The Yoga of Eating* p . 41-47 (chapter 7 The Central Practice).
3   Clark, N. (2014) *Sports Nutrition Guidebook (5ᵗʰ ed.)* Champaign, Illinois: Human Kinetics, p . 122 (p . 111-135 as resource on carbohydrates).

storage capacity; the more you train while well-fueled the greater your capacity. Example: an untrained runner may only have enough glycogen for 30 minutes of moderate activity and a few sprints while a well-trained athlete who fuels properly, regularly can have enough for up to three hours and several high intensity efforts. This depends on muscle fiber type, proper training and ablity to utilize oxygen and therefore fat as fuel source to conserve glycogen.[1] (There are many articles and thoughts on fat as fuel. I encourage you to read and learn as it applies to your training and experience.) On efforts lasting more than 60 minutes, consuming calories will fend off overtraining syndrome, prolong our stamina[2] and help maintain a higher level of performance. All of these factors have helped personalize my run nutrition plan as well as my recovery plan.

If our stomachs process 200–400 calories/hour while on the move, that means at a minimum I aim to consume at least two gels per hour or a package of Clif Bloks or an average energy bar. To give you an idea of calorie count, a quick list of my favorite pre-packaged energy foods are listed in the Fuel Chart, EXTRA PIECES page 224. It often baffles people how much they should consume.

If you have witnessed an aid station at the later stages of a 100-mile race, you have likely seen people down slices of pizza, handfuls of potatoes, burritos, peanut butter and jelly sandwiches, cups of soup, cola and countless other items likely exceeding the upper end of the estimated 200–400 per hour suggestion. In my experience, there comes a point of desired satiation, and eating something that resembles a meal is comforting amidst the countless gels and chewy things that have kept me going to that point. Sometimes this heavy aid station consumption comes with the consequence of having to move a bit slower for a few minutes. During that time, I visualize the meal as a lump of coal burning in my belly that will energize and fuel my later miles. To me, that satisfaction of being somewhat sated pays dividends as I approach the finish.

Choosing what to eat is part one. Timing and training yourself to eat is the more important part two. Because of our body's ability to use stored energy sources, you can run up to two hours (even three—think of top performing marathoners who are highly trained and super efficient—they are able to finish with a few sips of water or energy drink) without needing to consume calories while running. This changes as you prepare for longer distance training runs and races. You need to prepare yourself to be able to consume. For example: In my experience, the need for calorie intake starts with runs lasting longer than 90 minutes. This does not mean that I start taking calories at 90 minutes. This means that if I plan to run longer than 90 minutes, I consume at regular (20–30 minute) intervals from the beginning of the run.

To learn what to eat and when, it is helpful to test products and timing on your training runs. Work with a variety of product combinations. Learn when you can squeeze in more calories and when you need to back off. I aim to avoid palette fatigue and my strategy is to frontload. I consume the higher end of possible calories from whole foods and calorically dense products (potatoes, salted avocados, Trail Butter and First Endurance Ultragen recovery drink) early in the run/race and maintain this higher consumption for as long as I can. As the miles add up, my desire to eat decreases. That is when I switch to easier calories, like gels and Clif Bloks. Some people can ingest gels every 20 minutes for hours. I tend to fare better with variety.

It is also a good idea to introduce nutrition during your shorter runs, simply for the sake of adjusting your body to consume calories at regular intervals. Something to think about: You are burning calories while you are running. You have to replace them at some point to recover. Ingesting calories and hydrating during your run leaves you less behind on this process than if you consumed nothing. My point is that it will not hurt to consume gel or an energy drink on a 60–90 minute run and it will teach your body to consume earlier.

1 Clark, N. (2014) *Sports Nutrition Guidebook (5th ed.)* p. 196-201 Champaign, Illinois: Human Kinetics
2 Cooper, Dr. Emily Seattle Performance Medicine. Offered edits 4/2/15. Author summarized 5/14/15.

In 15 years of ultrarunning, my race day nutrition continues to evolve. What started as snacking from the standard aid station fare of peanut butter and jelly wedges, Clif Bars, potatoes dipped in salt, pretzels and bananas, evolved to a personalized crew serving up Trail Butter filled medjool dates, avocados with salt, First Endurance Ultragen recovery drink mid-race, gels and Clif Bloks. This menu will continue to evolve. I have learned that just when I think I have my nutrition plan dialed, it changes.

* For tips on carrying these products while on the run, see the Gear chapter, page 183 for Hydration Packs and/or Bottles.

Recovery Windows. 30-Minute Window. 90-Minute Window. And More!

Endurance sports push the human body to its outer limits. Since we are unable to consume as much as we burn while in motion, most of our longer training efforts will result in a calorie deficit—even if you consume the suggested maximum (400 calories/hour). It is extremely important to fuel sufficiently before, during and after your workouts in order to replenish and recover. Skipping this process or insufficiently fueling can create performance deficits, lead to overtraining syndrome and increase risk of injury.

When we finish a long run, or after an especially high-output workout, the body is in high demand and willing to receive and utilize what you consume for its recovery. You have two opportunities and need to take advantage of both. For the first 30 minutes after finishing your workout, the door to replenishing your muscle glycogen stores is wide open. It is easy to get caught up in conversation at the trailhead or to check your phone. I encourage you to make recovery your priority. Thirty minutes will disappear quickly and the door will slam shut[1] if you don't make the most of it. Avoid the phone, but you can keep the chatter going if you are with friends; just multi-task. Depending on the temperature and conditions, you might need to change into dry clothes to keep the body heat you earned. Or conversely, if it is hot, get out of the sun, rinse off your salty face and quickly move to step two: Hydrate (remember the Sweat Rate Test, you need to replace water/electrolytes too) and recovery nutrition.

There is an amazing amount of science and products available to help our bodies recover. Ingesting your calories using the generally accepted ratio of 3:1 (sometimes 4:1) carbohydrates to protein will help the body resynthesize muscle glycogen (carbs) and assist in muscle fiber regeneration. You can make this snack as simple or complex as you desire. Real food works. Pre-fabricated drinks work. There are studies that chocolate milk will get the job done. My mentor, Scott Jurek—a vegan, seven-time winner of the Western States 100, author of *Eat & Run* and a legend in our sport—once told me that, "something is better than nothing," when I had a couple of Red Vines and a Snickers bar from Halloween in my car after our unexpected long run. These definitely were not proper recovery, and fortunately I learned from this experience to be better stocked wiith good and plentiful nutrition to aid my recovery. Now, my body is dialed to my recovery routine. As I approach the final miles of a long run, I crave First Endurance Ultragen recovery drink. I prefer the convenience of this product (Fuel Chart page 224) and the science put in to it to ensure that I get what I need in that first 30-minute window.

Playing with these recovery windows, I have found that if I execute the first with a recovery drink I then have a little breathing room to head home, shower and prepare a meal to land in the second window about 1–3 hours post run. The timing typically works well. Just as the meal makes it on to my plate, my stomach

---

1   There is another theory that you have up to 90 minutes for your recovery window

starts to growl and I feel hungry again as if my muscles are telling me they are ready for more nutrients to continue the rebuilding process. Note: The number of these windows varies depending on the duration of exercise. Your recovery and replenishment will continue, listen to your body and continue to fuel appropriately.

Then there is the reality of life. What about when you've squeezed in your long run and you have to hurry home to jump back into child care or to start a work shift? In this instance it is even more important to listen to your body, otherwise you will be distracted from your recovery process. Have preplanned calories available and consume them within your recovery windows. Prepare the night before or plan a stop on the way back to reality to pick up something. Use this little mantra to help prioritize: *Something is better than nothing. Quantity over quality. Quality over convenience.* Do not justify a fast-food stop as your something. Instead, make a nut butter and jelly sandwich and bring an apple or banana. Pack leftovers from a healthy dinner the night before. Make good choices for your training. The overall goal is to kick-start recovery with immediate refueling, and then to follow up with further nutritional support after a couple of hours.[1]

After a long race or training run, people complain of (or revel in) being hungry for weeks. Something to consider: An athlete burns on average 800 calories per hour while running. During the course of 100 miles, the athlete might move for 20–30 hours. Do the math: 800 calories x 20 hours = 16,000 calories to 800 calories x 30 hours = 24,000 calories. Even if the athlete consumed 300 calories an hour, there is a (16,000-[300x20]) = 10,000 to (24,000-[300x30]) = 15,000 calorie deficit. Prior to the long effort you can pre-fuel a portion of the deficit calories because the likelihood of being able to replenish the debt soon after is slim. This is good idea especially if you plan to resume training right away. After the race it might take a while to replenish those depleted calories in addition to your increased metabolism and average daily requirement. Listen to your body, eat at frequent intervals and be prepared with healthy snacks.

Core and Strength

It is my opinion that the most common injuries for runners attempting longer distances are overuse injuries. Increasing mileage, while using the same muscle groups repetitively, puts increased stress on the system. This may challenge the body's ability to maintain performance without suffering some type of trauma. As you begin to adjust to the mileage increase and you improve your body's endurance, it is helpful to recruit stabilizing muscle groups to support your structure through the running motion. To remain strong and injury free, it is important to complement your running miles with core and strength work and cross-training.

---

1   Quoted from reference: http://training-conditioning.com/2010/04/17.the_recovery_window/index.php

Alternative **cardio** (no or little impact) exercises can help improve and maintain your fitness if the running miles are taking a toll on your body. Cycling, swimming, aqua jogging and elliptical training are all examples of other workouts to incorporate to maintain fitness. You can substitute cardio for "easy" mileage days or add it for extra low-impact endurance training.

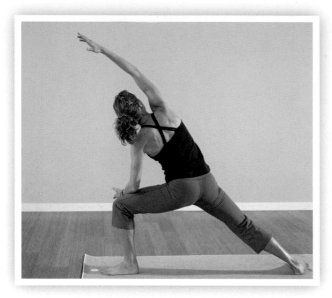

High school weight lifting class taught me to love the gym. Good form and techniques on basic and Olympic lifts helped familiarize and make me comfortable to execute a strength workout. Over time, working with physical therapists and doctors, I have learned more running-specific strength exercises. However you find your way to the important strength factor of training, I hope you make it a priority. Individuals will either enjoy or despise their non-running workouts. Finding respect for the strength cross-training gives you will keep you engaged and less prone to injuries. Specifically, recruiting and training muscles that are conducive to running is the goal.

To me, the most important forms of in-season cross-training are exercises that emphasize strength and flexibility. We strengthen the stabilizing muscles to support our larger muscle groups, ligaments, tendons and joints. We also work to turn these muscles on and get them to fire while running. Plenty of runners use their quadriceps and hamstrings, but minimally (or not at all) engage their gluteus. Strengthening and engaging these muscles will provide better stability to your running stride and reduce overuse injuries.

Utilizing our strength to gain flexibility maintains the importance of both in our injury prevention goal. Regular **stretching** (elongating movements), or in my case enlisting a **yoga** practice, engages my strength to encourage flexibility. Flexibility is different for everyone; my basic goal is to keep muscles long, the fibers fluid and well aligned. Flexibility, to me, is proper alignment and lengthening our muscles through movements opposite to running. I may never do the splits, but this does not mean I am not flexible relative to my starting point. In fact, I was told by my physical therapist that my body is tighter than average for females, but in the next breath said that this might contribute to my minimal injury and longevity because my joints are well supported. Appreciating my rigid body and working to maintain fluid and counter to running movement is my flexibility goal. I attribute my longevity in the sport to weekly yoga classes and can relate injuries to periods of high mileage, coupled with minimal stretching and strengthening. Improving and maintaining strength and flexibility leads to better running form and fewer injuries.

In 2005, I ran the Grand Slam of Ultrarunning, four 100-mile races in 11 weeks. My knees, specifically the underside of my kneecaps, were tender and painful by the last race. Afterwards, to aid in my recovery, I incorporated one-legged squats on a Bosu ball to strengthen my medial quad muscle and counter the pulling of my lateral quad. Balancing the strength in my quads alleviated my patella tendonitis. This exercise remains key in my weekly routine to maintain equal strength in the important quad muscles. Performing the repetitions while standing on a Bosu ball recruits and engages more stabilizing muscles.

For each gym exercise listed in my suggested training plans (page 45), I have a story of where I learned it, why I continue to incorporate it into my routine and my reason for recommending it to you. During your training plan, you will see a minimum of two days of core strength exercise work per week. To fulfill these you can work with the exercises and suggested routines. If you need more support, hire a personal trainer to dial in a strength program and help you with form. If motivation is your hold up, test out group exercise classes.

I encourage you to enlist strength/flexibility programs that work for you and more importantly, that you will do. Enjoyment is a key part of fitness and it is important to me that you thrive in these sessions as much as you revel in your running. Runners love to run. A lot of times that is all we want to do. Strive to make these workouts a part of your training that you look forward to, you are comfortable with and that you feel the benefits of in your running.

Power Hiking

Running long distances in the mountains often requires a variety of paces, and I think it is important to specifically train in power hiking so that you can make the most of the steeper sections of your race course, assuming you've chosen a mountainous course. It is also a good idea to take advantage of power hiking on lesser climbs to give your running muscles and mind a break. When training your power hiking skills on your hill workout days, make sure your effort level is high. You may be walking instead of running, but on a hill you can definitely push your heart rate by moving with intention.

When power hiking, I first think about the transition from running to hiking. Do not stop or slow down. Keep your momentum. I either swing my arms a bit more aggressively to encourage a faster hiking pace, or push my hands off of my knees for leverage. It is a good idea to keep your eyes and chest up and look ahead on the trail. Decide when you are going to start running again so that you do not get stuck in a walking pace. Looking and planning ahead helps you keep a more upright posture. Do not bend at the hips or slouch when power hiking. On some courses (Hardrock 100) you may be power hiking for an hour or more, so be sure to keep after the effort and look for the opportunity to run again, even if it is only for a few strides. When you transition back to running quicken your turnover, push off from your feet and make it as smooth as possible.

Night Running

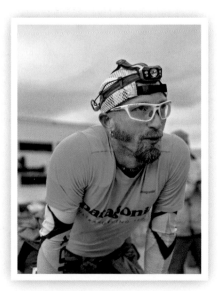

If there is a chance you will run through the dark during your race, most likely in races 50 miles or longer, you should definitely train in the dark evening or nighttime hours. Early pre-dawn hours will work as well. Running in the dark is tricky for two, or possibly three, key reasons. First, in nighttime hours our bodies are accustomed to the need for sleep, and we fight fatigue. Second, limited or no light makes it impossible to see anything, let alone the obstacles of trail running. Third, for some, is the fear of the dark.

To train and hopefully avoid sleep monsters—the overwhelming drowsy feeling that crawls up your spine, causes your eyes to close and your body to slow down—during your race, incorporate night running into your training. I find it easiest to start in the early evening and run at least thirty minutes before sunset and move into the night, as you will in your race. Adjust your clothing to accommodate for temperature shifts and fiddle with your lights before the sun disappears to prepare for the ensuing darkness. Consider nutrition options as a way to help fight off fatigue. Caffeinated

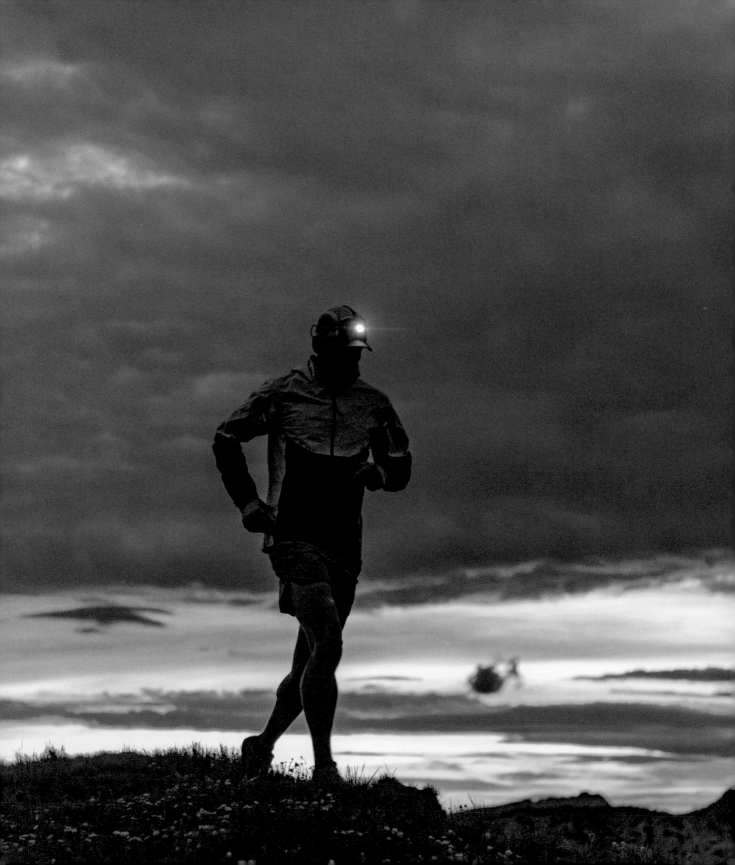

Pacing Darcy Piceu at the Hardrock 100 is perhaps my favorite dawn story. We had run through the night and she was literally falling asleep as we hiked up Grants Swamp Pass. We had less than 20 miles to the finish and mid-conversation she would stop responding, and I would look back to see her hunched over her poles. When the sun finally peered over Oscar's Pass behind us, I stopped in front of her pulled out a caffeinated gel and grabbed her shoulders to turn and face her towards the sun. The glow lit up her face as she consumed the mocha-flavored gooeyness. She blinked her eyes a few times, looked me square in the face and said, "Alright. I'm awake. Let's finish this *f'ing* thing." She won. Proud of that girl.

gels or even consuming a few extra calories right at sunset might give you a glycogen burst and help trigger alertness. Alternatively, you can start running 30–60 minutes before sunrise. The awakening that dawn provides is an experience in and of itself.

For me, running from 2 a.m.–4 a.m. is the most difficult time to stay awake. I am not suggesting that you train at 2 a.m.–4 a.m., but I'm offering this tidbit to bring awareness to the possible tough time period. These early morning hours are typically the coldest and darkest and feel the furthest from the hope of daylight. Prepare with warm clothing options, good lights and even a talkative pacer to help make those hours pass. Right before the sun comes up is typically when I feel like there is no possible way I will finish. But then, those first few golden rays are like magic.

It is important to figure out your lighting system. This is important for navigating the obstacles and staying on course. As you turn your training runs to a few nighttime adventures, be sure to fidget with the battery pack, learn the dimming capabilities to save battery life and play with head strap adjustments and waist belt attachment options. Look into varied colored lights (white, green or red are the most common) and discern if one or a combination of functions is better for your eyes. Utilize two lights to create a better depth of field. (See page 184 in the Gear chapter for product recommendations.)

I prefer to wear one light on my waist and to hold one in my hand. Typically I use a headlamp and extend the strap to its full extent to fit around my hips. I push it down on my pelvis to make the light more stable. I rarely turn the waist lamp off. I also carry one in my hand that I turn on only when moving quickly downhill. This allows me to point the light in the direction I want, scan ahead or augment the light from my waist. Often times I use another headlamp looped around my wrist for that second light so that my hands are free for eating or drinking. More light is better. The more you can see the faster you can run.

Finally, if you have a fear of the dark, nighttime running might be the biggest mental obstacle in your ultra race preparation. I suggest training with friends and creating safe experiences so that you feel comfortable moving into the darkness. Running early in the morning (predawn) gives you the confidence that you are moving into light. You know the sun will rise in an hour or two, depending on when you start, and it is a good way to first adjust to running in dark hours. I also encourage you to train a few evening runs; it is smart to be well-situated with your timing, when to pull out your lights, gear up and eat as you move into darkness. The more opportunities you have to test your lights and to be comfortable with your system, the more enjoyable night running will be. Be extra prepared with a backup light, fresh batteries, an extra jacket, beanie, gloves and a few extra calories. Preparation will help you feel more secure.

More light is better, unless you are **competing**. There have been a few times running under a full moon that my pacer has told me to turn off my lights. With just enough moonlight on the smooth path, we were able to zoom along the trail away from competition or sneak up on runners ahead. The idea being that you can't chase what you can't see, so if the competition can't see (my lights) they won't push as hard to chase me down. Likewise, if runners ahead are looking over their shoulder and they don't see me, they might ease their pace giving me and my late race surge, a chance at moving up in the field. This is just something to keep in mind while dancing around in the dark and the fun game might help keep you awake too.

Sleep Deprivation Training

Some people feel it is important to train your system to learn to live without sleep. I am not one of those people. It seems to me that there are plenty of opportunities in life where I have to push through something without enough sleep that I know what it feels like. I don't like it. When it comes to training and racing, I feel that the more rested you are, the better your body will recover. The more rested you are going into a race, the more you can draw from in those wee morning hours. Think of your sleep as a bank account. Each night you get a good night sleep or afternoon when you sneak in a nap, you are making a deposit in the sleep account. When you spend long days awake or miss a night's sleep, you withdraw. There is no doubt you are going to withdraw on race day/night, so I feel it is best to have a large sum to pull from when that day comes. Do not force yourself to live without your precious rest. Instead, when your life is challenging and a good night's sleep is where you have to give, then you can think of it as sleep deprivation training.

Time on Feet

Running for two–three hours early on a Sunday morning, stopping for a latte and landing on the Seattle Running Company floor by 9:50 a.m. was a pretty common routine to wrap up my week of classes at the University of Washington. In my early ultra days I convinced myself, with calves slashed with mud, that time on feet was a good way to train for an ultra. Ten to 15 miles first thing in the morning followed by a six to eight hour workday was a bit of an ultra in itself, if anything for the mental training.

One major difference I have witnessed in ultra training plans versus marathon training plans is **back-to-back** long runs for ultras, where marathon training plans tend to have one long run a week sandwiched by two lower mileage days. The back-to-back long runs, typically scheduled over the weekends, teach you to run on tired legs. The recovery between the runs is important for refueling and sleeping. Getting out again after the first long day will simulate the later stages of an ultra and show you that you can run even when you are tired. Also it is highly unlikely that you will run 70-80 percent of your distance in training like you would in a marathon, it would be difficult to recover from. Therefore, the back-to-back runs are a good way to prepare your body for your ultra race.

I still subscribe to time on feet and back-to-back training, and while recovery becomes more important as my miles and years add up, I believe long days and utilizing the realities of life to help you train for your ultra are beneficial.

Preventing Issues

Perhaps the most important trick of the trade is learning to anticipate and prevent debilitating situations. Take care of the little things before they become big things. This applies to clothing, gear, blisters, hydration and nutrition. . . basically everything. The only way to know what works and what does not work for you is to practice and dial in all of your systems so that each functions in a variety of circumstances and situations.

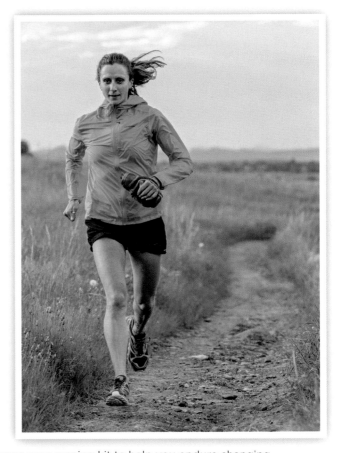

Weather is perhaps the best example in preparation. You must manage your core body temperature, whether in the blistering heat of the day or through frigid nights. The energy you burn shivering to keep warm on a chilly night can be the difference between a finish or a DNF. This exact situation lead to my 2011 DNF at the Ultra Trail du Mont Blanc. Do not tough it out in a t-shirt and shorts on a 40°F rainy day. If you are starting to chafe or blister, add Body Glide or change clothes/socks before it is an issue. Wear the right layers to keep your body dry, friction-free and warm, but not overheating. During the course of an ultra, you may need to adjust, add to or completely change your running kit to help you endure changing conditions. Stay aware and plan ahead. Watch the sky for building clouds or check weather reports for possible heat waves or storms.

As temperatures climb your body may not respond to the fuel options you trained with and you may not want to eat. Altitude and travel may also throw off your system. Tune-in and take care to continue eating and drinking. You will have to adjust the quantities and timing, just ensure you contiue fueling. Cooling your core with ice around your neck and down your back (sports bra on women is ideal!) may also encourage your appetite. Do not force anything but work to get your system back on track. Fueling is a key component to your training and racing, I hope you can avoid this being a major issue.

Finally, carry a few extra items for the just-in-case scenario. (I always carry a beanie, my Houdini jacket—the lightweight Patagonia jacket that has literally saved my life five times—gloves and an extra Clif Bar—more calories than I think I need—for any run over two hours, always.) Execute in anticipation and be aware of the conditions and your body to avoid having to fix complicated or irreversible situations.

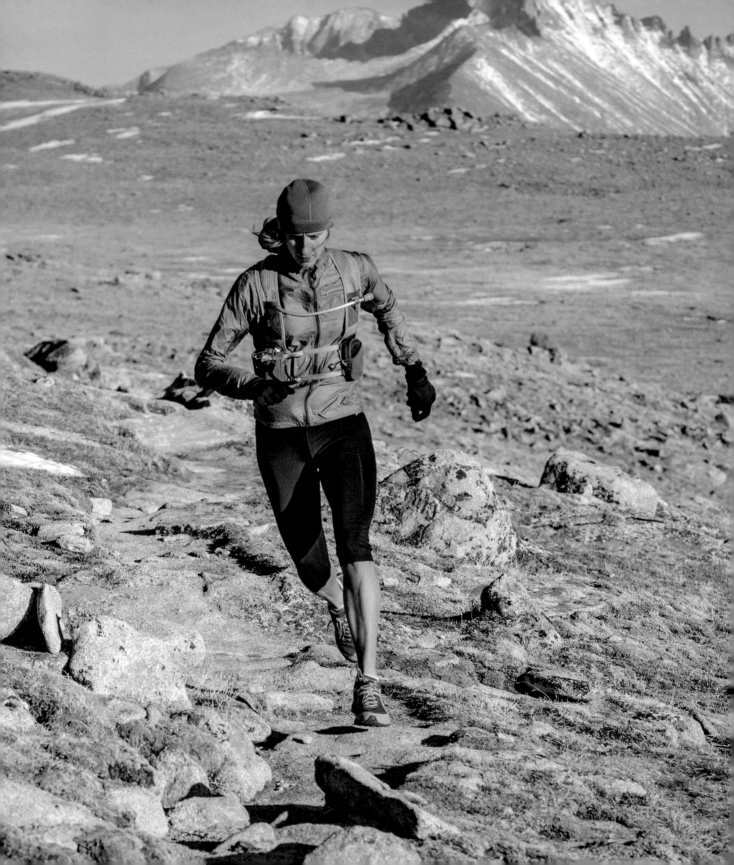

TRAIN YOUR BRAIN

Training for an ultra is very physical. You have a training plan that maps out your miles and core training. You have gear to test, mentors to engage, books and online resources to devour. There are coaches, psychologists, loved ones and friends who can help you to see what you have deep down inside; they can tell you what it takes to push through the challenge. But to truly learn it, you have to go through it and see yourself come out the other side of what seemed impossible. Finishing an ultra is (arguably) 100 percent mental.

The *what-ifs, I can't's and I should haves*. There are many sentences that start with these phrases and they will likely run through your mind at various stages of training and racing. They bring up doubt and uncertainty. They are also your opportunity to train your brain. It takes mental strength to answer these questions with confidence, and that strength will see you through to the ultra finish line. This mental training becomes more important as the distance of your goal increases. Each long training run and race will teach you about your limits and your ability to challenge mental boundaries. Most people do not realize the importance of the mental side until they reach the finish line.

These tips will help you train your brain by raising awareness to potential upcoming challenges. I aim to trigger your internal drive, to keep you going when times are rough and to give you a glimmer of what is necessary, before you toe the start line.

VISUALIZATION

For my first 100-mile race, I bit off much more than I ever recommend to a newbie 100-mile runner. I wanted to be the youngest and the fifth woman in the race's 24-year history to break 24 hours at the Wasatch Front 100-mile race. In making this goal I prepared like no other newbie I knew. I quizzed previous champions on how they trained. I put in quality training miles and raced myself into shape all summer in preparation for the fall 100. I previewed the mountains in training runs with locals and I enlisted an experienced crew. All of these pieces added up to an amazing race day, but I believe the piece that made me believe I could do it was visualization.

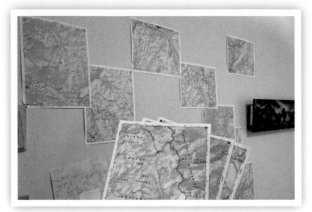
Maps for the John Muir Trail FKT covered my bedroom wall for four months.

When my entry to the Wasatch Front 100 was accepted in January, I printed off the course description and read a section nearly every night for the next nine months. If I didn't have my papers with me, I would recall as much as I could. After I spent time running on the course, I matched the visuals from my training runs to my readings of the course description. As the race approached I placed myself into the visualizations. I sunk deep into my body to know exactly how I would feel climbing Chinscraper 18 miles in. I felt the sun on my face and the heat surrounding my body climbing out of Alexander Springs. My hands felt sticky pushing off my quads climbing up Catherine's Pass. I felt the trail reverberating in my legs as I descended into Pot Bottom. I could see Clif Bar remnants on Roch's mustache as my pacer talked me through the last climb. I thought about and over-thought what race day would be like. I sent myself on to that course many times throughout the spring and summer, whether lying in bed or while running through the Cascades. Every training effort focused on how it would impact my Wasatch.

Suggestions:

➜ Pin maps up on a wall to look at every day.

➜ Read through sections of the course description at least once a week. More frequently as you get closer to the event.

➜ Preview the course and lock in visuals of the trail.

➜ Listen to others tell their stories about the race. Hopefully someone that is a good, descriptive storyteller.

➜ Gather as much information as possible by reading the website thoroughly, and reviewing detailed blog posts and articles about the race.

➜ While training, visualize the miles you are running as miles on the course. Project how you want to feel at mile 55, mile 82 and mile 98.

RACE MENTALITY

When you first picked up this book or decided to run an ultra, there was a spark, a bit of internal excitement that put you over the edge to make you decide to execute on the idea. Dig back to that first interest. Hold on to that spark through your training and into your race. That desire to know the unknown is a huge motivator. It will keep you humble and curious. It will remind you of the respect you have for the distance and the training you have to endure. On race day, that spark will spread like fire through your body as you are finally executing and peering into that unknown.

As the race approaches, depending on your personality, there is potential for nervous energy to take over. Acknowledge it and view it as respect for the distance you are about to tackle. I now know that if I am not nervous for a race then I should not be standing on the start line. There should be some excitement and wonderment that causes that bubbly feeling inside. Keeping calm and not wasting energy is the confidence I hope you build through your training. When the nerves speak up, breathe and take confidence in your training. Harness the nervous energy and excitement and visualize it as a pocket of energy that you can dig into later.

Race mentality has different meanings to each person. I have seen people retreat, completely internally, and show up at the start line presumably out of nowhere. I have witnessed the familiar bubbly type that nonchalantly socializes taking in the whole experience. There are others that run around buying last-minute aids, thinking it will help them to the finish, question everyone in sight about how they should run their race, pack and repack their drop bags and fret about what to eat for dinner. It may come as no surprise that in 15 years of running I have portrayed each of these prerace jitter personalities at different events, and it is likely that you will too.

The good thing about reading through these now is that you have a choice. You get to decide how you want your prerace routine to unfold. Make a plan, share it with your crew, be flexible for snags that may arise and plan accordingly to alleviate any possible deterrents from your plan.

Spreading the Peanut Butter

The following is an interpretation of an analogy told by my good friend and training partner, Roch Horton.

All of your training is peanut butter. Yes, you read that right: I am equating your training to nut butter. When you start training, you have an empty jar. All season you fill that jar with workouts and long runs, recovery periods and rest, good nutrition and practice races. Every effort you make in preparation for your goal race is more peanut butter to fill the jar.

As training wraps up and you move into the taper for your "A" race, (the focus, goal race that you have trained for all year) that is when it is time to take inventory. How much training have you done? How full is the jar? The next question is; how will you use it on race day? My friend Roch's peanut butter analogy might be the ticket to help you plan your race day and may just make you hungry for it (the race and peanut butter).

The course of your goal race is toast, a piece of bread hot out of the toaster.

The knife is your execution, running the event. When the gun fires, your knife holds every ounce of peanut butter stored for this race.

Now you have a decision. How are you going to spread the peanut butter? You have one swipe, one opportunity to spread the peanut butter over this piece of toast. Are you going to load the front corner with the majority? Will you spread it thin up front and heavy toward the back? Or will you spread it out evenly over the piece of toast? If you put it all down up front, then it will look pretty thin toward the end. If you aim to spread evenly, will you end up with too much at the finish?

Now substitute your energy for the peanut butter. How are you going to spread it?

This story was also published on the Ultraspire Blog: http://ultraspire.com/how-to-run-spread-the-peanut-butter/

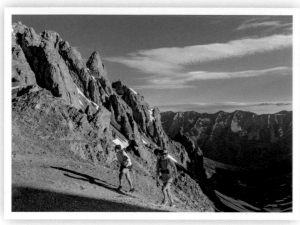

Pacing Daray Piceu to her Hardrock win, 2012

Suggestions:

➜ Make all travel plans well in advance.

➜ Book hotels, flights, cars.

➜ Plan race food and purchase a week in advance.

➜ Make a list of last-minute perishables and ask a crewmember to pick them up closer to race day.

➜ Write a tentative schedule for the days leading up to and following the race. This should be in addition to your race day time sheet (Race Time Sheet on page 228)

➜ Include travel times, grocery stops, food prep and goal bedtime.

Q&A: ANSWERS TO THE DOUBTS

If you find yourself worrying and doubting, check out this section. A few of the Q&A's may help dissolve your concerns.

1. AT THE START OF YOUR TRAINING:

Your thought: "I just can't fit a workout in. I'm tired after work. There is too much on my plate."

My advice: Acknowledge that starting any new endeavor is challenging. Making changes to our routine schedule is probably one of the most disruptive adjustments. This adjustment is testing your desire. Running an ultra sounded like a great idea when you bought this book. Now as the reality sets in, how much do you want this? I believe that if you turned to this chapter looking for this piece of advice, you really do want it. You are going through the hardest part, changing your schedule to incorporate the training. Once you get through this adjustment, (they say 21 days to "habit") this will flow much easier.

Tips to help find that flow:

➜ Before going to bed, plan your training block for the next day. Pack clothes, fuel, watch and everything you will need so that it is ready to go.

➜ If scheduling is an issue, with family or work, let the important people of your life know when you plan to run/train. Double-check that your plan works with their schedule and, if appropriate, ask for their encouragement to put you out the door.

2. AS YOU START THE 3RD WEEK DURING A TOUGH BUILDING PHASE:

Your thought: "I pushed hard in week two and there is still another big week ahead! Logging the miles scheduled seems a bit daunting. I am wavering in my enthusiasm." This can be the case especially if life is adding additional time constraints making the training time harder to fit in.

My advice: First check in with the possibility of injury. Pushing through a workout when injury is creeping in is the last thing you want to do. How to know if you are injured? Is your running gait altered? Are you favoring the sore/tender spot? If you said yes to either of these, read through the injury prevention chapter (page 163).

If injury is not the issue and the resistance to the mileage comes from feeling tired or a lack of motivation, check in with what is causing these feelings. Are you getting enough sleep on a consistent basis? Are you fueling well? Are you hitting your recovery windows? (See Tricks of the Trade-Recovery Windows page 24). Is additional life stress distracting you from your training focus? As you address these questions you will understand your resistance. Acknowledging the cause will help you process and get back to your training.

Tips for motivating:

→ If life stress is the issue, utilize your running as *your* break from it all, the thing you do for you. Do not view your running as another stressor piling on your system. Likewise, do not use your run to escape, instead let your brain process and move through some of the day-to-day stressors. My quote: There are not many issues in life a long run can't solve. It's just that sometimes the run needs to be a bit longer.

→ If you are physically fatigued and on the verge of burnout, either move the schedule around to take an easy day or completely skip a workout. (Do not try to work it in later in the week.) Knowing that you have the ability to manage your training will help with your motivation.

→ If you are not sleeping well or having a hard time going to sleep, check in on your training time and caffeine intake. As we increase our training load, especially if workouts are done later in the day, it can be difficult to sleep at night. Run in the morning or early afternoon so that your body has time to process the endorphins and wind down before bed. Caffeine consumed later in the day can also impact your sleeping patterns.

→ If your lack of motivation is more serious, check out the burnout section in the Injury Prevention chapter on page 165.

3. AS YOU START A RECOVERY WEEK:

Your thought: "The schedule says an easy five miles, but (insert one of the following: "it's cold outside," "the day got away from me," "I don't want to tie my shoes," "I didn't eat right," "I didn't sleep well last night," or whatever other reason you have) and I just don't feel like it."

My advice: Rest. Make a conscious decision to skip the run, make a note on your calendar to remind yourself why you made this decision and happily rest so that this is a positive decision. Do not make up the easy five miles. My hope and plan during recovery weeks is to recharge your body and mind. If your mind is fighting you just to get out the door for an easy five miles, then it is time to rest. By giving yourself this break your training desire will return. You will need it as we pick up the weekly mileage again in the next build phase. Finally, do not feel guilty for it.

4. 1–2 WEEKS OUT FROM YOUR RACE.

Your thought: "Have I done enough training? Am I really ready for this race? What about that one week I had a cold and couldn't do half of the workouts."

My advice: If you have done 70–80 percent of the training, I really think you are ready. It is okay to question. The nerves building and questioning your training are signs of respect for the challenge that you are about to undertake. This is where good notes in your calendar will help. Look back over some of your higher mileage weeks and solid building phases. Note the ones where you felt strongest. Read through those notes to yourself and feel confident in your training.

Your thought: "I think I should run more. I have plenty of time and it's just killing me to be tapering right now."

My advice: This frustration and agitated state is also known as Taper Tantrums. Your body is strong and well tuned to your consistent schedule. It might feel like it is craving more work than what you are giving it during your taper. This feeling is a good thing. Ten days to two weeks out from your race, the taper phase, is the final part to your overall periodization.[1] The building blocks you have worked through (three weeks building, one week recovery) are now are a part of a bigger building block culminating in your race performance. The energy building inside is your body responding to your training plan; it is recovering and integrating your training. Consistency remains key, noting that a reduction in volume and intensity has shown improved distance running performance and running economy.[2]

During your taper think about what you can do. Use all of this excess energy to visualize and organize for your race. If you find yourself buzzing around wasting energy, focus it.

→ Relax in a comfortable chair with a warm beverage and read through the course description or a race report. Close your eyes and visualize how you want to feel at various points on the course. Think about pacing. Will you hike the hills? Strategize how quickly you will move through aid stations. If this is your first 50k and you have completed a marathon distance (either in a race or training), imagine what you want to feel like at mile 28. Visualize your strong finish. Who will be there cheering you on as you cross the line? Do the best you can to tune into what you want to feel like in each of these moments.

→ Pack your bags. A week out may seem early, but the weekend before your race you will have some extra time. You should not be running long, so why not create some ease in the coming week. Pack your race bag. (See Race Packing List page 226 for tips on what to include.) As you pack, make a list of any items you still need to pick up so that you can purchase them early in the week rather than raiding a 24-hour convenience store the night before the race.

→ **Make a meal.** Suggested menus to right. Have a few friends over, keep it simple and cook everyone a great dinner or brunch. Find ease with this process; enjoy the planning, shopping and preparation. As people arrive, enjoy sitting down and catching up. Avoid talking about your race. Make a point of catching up with these friends. If your race comes up in conversation, focus on what you are looking forward to and what you hope to gain from the experience. Telling these positive stories will continue to add to your race day. Having caught up with friends will give your mind fun things to think about while you are on the trail.

---

1   Katch VL, McArdle WD, Katch Fl. *Essentials of Exercise Physiology* (4th ed.) (2006). Baltimore, MD: Lippincott, Williams & Wilkins. p. 472.
2   Houmard, J.A., Scott, L.S., Justice, C.L. and Chenier, T.C. (1994). The effects of taper on performance in distance runners. *Medicine and Science in Sports and Exercise. 26(5),* 624-31.

Stir fry dinner menu and shopping list:

→ 2 cups (380 g) rice (I prefer Basmati)
→ 2–4 tablespoons (30–60 ml) coconut or olive oil
→ 1 white onion
→ 3–6 cloves of garlic, pressed

→ 1–2" fresh ginger, peeled and grated
→ 1 pound (450 g) protein (chicken, sausage, tofu, beef, seafood)
→ 3 bell peppers (red, yellow and orange)

You can choose from the following or get creative at the farmers' market or grocery store:

→ Sugar snap peas
→ Broccoli crowns

→ Purple cabbage
→ Mushrooms

I like the basic flavor of the vegetables, but feel free to experiment with sauces (For example: peanut, soy, tamari, curry paste, Sriracha). Add sauce as a final touch with the vegetables.

Add the rice with four cups (950 ml) of water to a rice cooker. Cut all vegetables into large, bite-size pieces (about 1-2 inches [2.5-5 cm], chunks or slices). Sauté the onion, garlic and ginger in oil on medium-low heat until the onions are translucent. Add the protein and cook through. Add the remaining vegetables and sauce, then cook until al dente. Serve over cooked rice.

Waffle or pancake bar brunch menu and shopping list:

Follow your favorite batter recipe or use a prepackaged mix (I like Bob's Redmill). Prepare enough and keep them warm in the oven.

Extras: bacon, scrambled eggs, fruit platter, coffee, hot tea, fresh squeezed orange juice.

Toppings for the bar: Prepare small bowls and create a fun buffet for your guests to top their waffles or pancakes.

→ Fresh berries
→ Sliced bananas
→ Maple syrup
→ Trail butter
→ Chocolate chips
→ Honey

→ Molasses
→ Yogurt
→ Butter
→ Seed mixtures
→ Cinnamon

* My favorite waffle toppers are plain Greek yogurt, maple syrup and Flora 7 Sources.

5. MID-RACE BLOW UP

This is a big one to come back from mentally. It is challenging to turn your mind around when your physical body is failing you and now you are sitting on a chair with your head between your knees, when you thought you would be cruising through the race miles.

Your thought: "I'm done. I can't eat. I feel nauseous. I threw up. My quads are worked. I feel dizzy. I can't run like I thought I would be running. I am (fill in the blank)."

My advice: Take a deep breath, look at your crew and smile. Try to take the seriousness out of your blow up. Maybe one of them can make you laugh or you can crack a joke that gets them laughing. Try, "I paid for this?" or "This is fun, right?" That last one is especially good right after you throw up. You will be amazed how smiling and laughing will change your perspective.

Give yourself a minute. As you take that deep breath, check in with yourself. All of your training has taught you to be in tune with your body. Ask yourself, "What do I need in this moment to feel better? Have I eaten enough? Am I hydrated? When was the last time I took electrolytes?" If it is hot, cooling your body down with ice around your neck, washing off your face and swallowing small ice chips will help reduce your core temperature. Taking the time to change your clothes, socks and even shoes can give you a renewed spirit. Perhaps your spirited crew will give you a leg rub to help those beat up quads. Walk out of the aid station and give yourself one more section to see if your body and mind will rally. You might run the second half faster than the first! You might settle into a rhythm that allows you to meet your goal. Crazier things have happened, and we learn the most about ourselves when we test our limits.

If laughing isn't an option, taking a break doesn't help, and this is more serious, I recommend checking in with the medical team. If you have not urinated in a couple of hours, your hands are swollen, your weight is up or down or other physical symptoms are adding to your blow up, it is a good idea to engage with a medical professional. Ideally, he/she has experience in the ultra world to understand what you are putting your body through and can help make smart decisions for your body.

Finally, if this is just a rough go (no serious medical issues at stake) and you are faced with walking it in or quitting, refer to your prerace plan (Race Day Preparations: Ready? Set?, Mentally and What If Question: DNF Plan, page 204). You made a decision about whether you would want to complete this no matter what or if you prefer to try again later. Be confident in your decision, either way.

6. AS YOU DEAL WITH AN INJURY

Your thought: I have consistent pain in my (fill in the blank). I feel like I can run through it, but I'm worried it will get worse.

My advice: Without being able to talk to you face-to-face, this is a tricky scenario. Listening to your body and not your desire is the key to knowing when to run and when to rest. When running, does the pain get worse? Does it hurt before and after, but not during? Does it only hurt during? Where exactly does it hurt? How does the pain present itself? Are there any other referring painful points? Often injuries are caused in one part of the chain, but present in another. Ex: IT Band Syndrome typically starts with weak and tight gluteus muscles, but presents as an ice pick stabbing the outside of your knee. Are there strengthening and stretching exercises you do that make it feel better? Finally, enlist the advice of a professional (physical therapist, doctor, etc.) to aid your decision.

Your thought: I know my body well enough and this pain/injury will turn into something bad if I don't take care of it now.

My advice: First of all, I am psyched that your awareness enables you to make this call for yourself. That deserves huge applause! Taking the time now to heal the injury will not only give you the chance to run your goal race, it will likely ensure your longevity in the sport as you approach a more sustainable mindset.

Second, focus your energy on your recovery. When injured, it is easy to stop everything because running isn't an option. It is better to use the time and energy to repair your body. Get a proper diagnosis from a professional so that you can heal the injury and create a recovery plan. As noted in the previous injury question, often the pain is the referral point and the actual issue is further along the chain. Be diligent about healing the area and return to training mindfully to ensure full recovery.

Your reality: Injury is serious and you are unable to run.

My advice: It happens and it sucks at first. (I just spent 15 minutes with the thesaurus trying to find a better word, but "sucks" really sums it up.) I am sure it feels like the worst possible time in your training plan and you are understandably incredibly bummed. Allow yourself to feel that; mad, sad whatever emotion comes up. Then focus on the bigger picture. There is more to your running goals than one race. Long-distance running is a lifestyle and to maintain your body's ability to manage your daily running endeavors, you

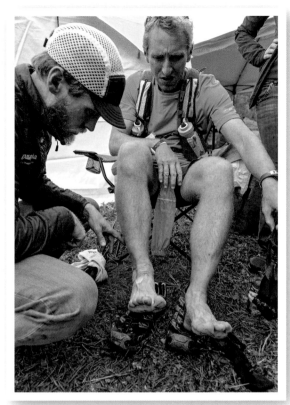

Luke Nelson steps in to help Hardrock runner Ryan McDermott diagnose and keep moving.

must take this opportunity to learn. What caused the injury? What might have prevented it? How can you incorporate these to avoid future injuries? Focus on your healing process. Put the time that you would have spent training into your rehabilitation.

Injury Recovery Workouts

Injury never comes at a good time and while some may want to discontinue any form of training, I encourage you to maintain your fitness and movement. Give your body everything it needs to repair this injury, including a correct diagnosis, treatment plan, nutrition, strength routine and daily focus on healing. It is worth obtaining a gym membership (you could try month-to-month) to give you access to machines and fitness classes.

The following are workout suggestions to keep your recovery creative and you motivated when running is not an option. These workouts do not have to be done in this order. You will likely need to move them around according to your treatment plan and the severity of your injury. You can add time and intervals as you improve. The goal is to have two workouts a week, and two to three endurance days a week. Rest days are still important—perhaps more important—during injury recovery.

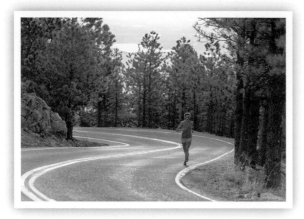

Suggestions:

WORKOUT 1:

Swim laps or aqua-jog, 30–50 minutes.

Enlist a pyramid or ladder workout to keep this interesting, whether you are swimming laps or aqua-jogging. Establish segments to work harder and segments to recover.

WORKOUT 2:

45–60 minutes on the elliptical.

Warm up and cool down about 10 minutes each. Maintain a steady effort for the remainder.

WORKOUT 3:

45–60 minutes on the elliptical. Core strength exercises.

Enlist a pyramid or ladder workout to keep the elliptical interesting. Establish segments to work harder and segments to recover. Knock out a second workout with a core strength exercise session and integrate key exercises to aid the recovery of your injury.

WORKOUT 4:

Spin class. Kickbox class. Aerobics class.

There are a variety of group exercise classes that will challenge your comfort zone as well as your fitness. As long as the movements do not aggravate your injury, I encourage this dynamic movement for fun, to engage different muscles and bring a new workout to your regimen. Who knows, you might like it and keep incorporating it even after you are healed!

WORKOUT 5:

15 minutes on the rowing machine, 15 minutes on the elliptical, 15 minutes on the stationary bike. Core strength exercises.

On each machine, warm up for the first 5 minutes. Push hard (think 5 minute interval workout effort) the middle 5–8 minutes, cool down the last 3–5 minutes. Move quickly to the next machine. Knock out a second workout with a core strength exercises session and integrate key exercises to aid the recovery of your injury.

WORKOUT 6:

90 minutes–2 hours

This involves endurance effort. You can break this up into two or three machines or swim laps, to keep it interesting. (Two hours is about my maximum time on machines. You can increase this time to improve your endurance if it is not crazy-making.)

Training Plan Adjustments: When restarting a training plan after injury, I encourage you to start during the recovery week. The lower mileage will allow you to ease back into the plan, test your structure and continue your injury recovery regime.

Suggestions:

→ If you take 2-3 weeks off from running to heal your injury, return to the training block from which you left. Ex: If you injured yourself and stopped running at week 10, restart with week 8, which is a recovery week from the previous block.

→ If you take 4-6 weeks off from training, restart with the previous training block. Ex: If you stop at week 15, restart with week 8.

→ If you take 2-3 months to recover, depending on your base, you can either restart the program or restart 2-3 building phases prior to where you left. Ex: If you stop at week 21, restart with week 8 or week 12.

→ If you take more than 3 months, you should consider restarting the program.

→ If your injury occurs during the last building phase or during your taper, rest. Receive massage. Ice. Heat. Do whatever the professionals tell you. Forget about the rest of your training and do everything to get yourself healthy by race day. Your ability to race will depend on the severity of your injury and how quickly you can fully heal it, but it is still possible even if you barely run the final 3-4 weeks prior to your race. Do not race if you are not fully healed.

7. DNF – Did Not Finish

Your reality: You started your race, but you did not finish.

My advice: Be confident in the decision you made. Know that this is a learning experience and not a measure of you. There will be emotions that come up. Feel them and move on. I encourage you not dwell on them. Quickly move beyond any negative thoughts and work toward understanding what happened. Evaluate your day soon after the event, write down your thoughts and then leave them aside for a couple of days. Focus on your recovery (race recovery chapter pg 207). Even though you did not finish, it is important to recover fully before jumping into another race goal. About a week later, revisit your DNF notes with a different perspective. Do you see the event differently? Was there a cause unrelated to your physical training (mental, emotional, weather, unexpected circumstance) that added to or instigated your stopping? Can you look into your training and find changes that might help you finish next time? Were there aspects of your preparation that were not as dialed as they could have been? Were you too focused on the goal and not enjoying the experience? Did you run faster than your planned pace? As you work through these answers, find your love of the sport, renew your motivation and allow yourself to dream about future goals. Your first finish will be even sweeter.

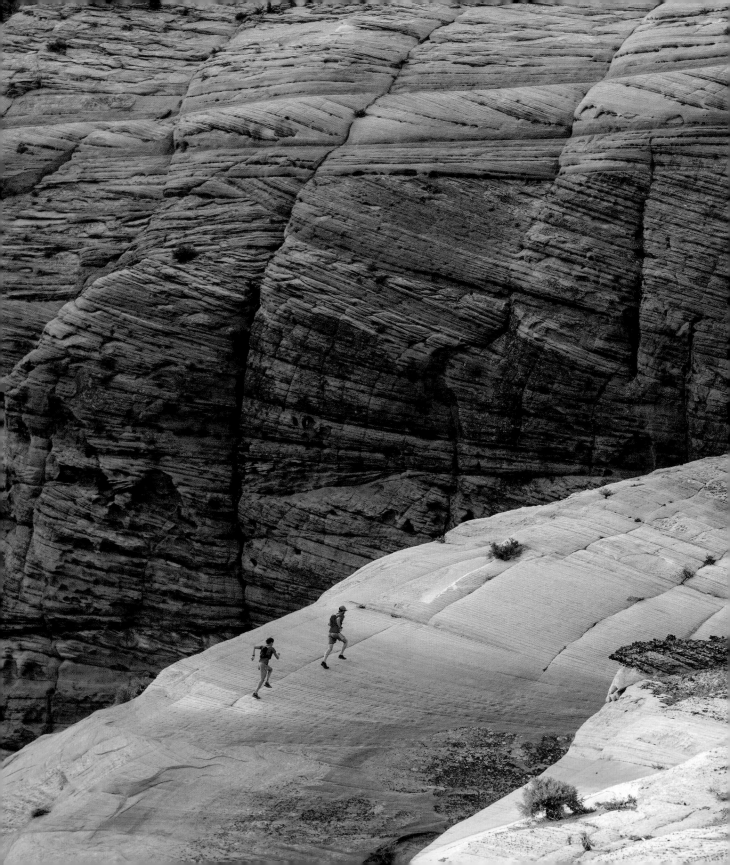

TRAINING PLANS

Variety is the spice of life. I want to keep you on your toes, engaged and enjoying your training. On the pages ahead, you will not see repetitive training plans. (Ex: Monday mid-mileage run and core, Tuesday interval workout, Wednesday rest, Thursday longer miles, Friday hills, Saturday long run, Sunday rest.) Instead, the weeks build on one another and workouts are strategically staggered to give you rest or push you as necessary. I hope you enjoy my method of changing up the weekly schedule to keep your body and mind engaged.

"While (Rickey) Gates doesn't subscribe to a hard-nosed training plan, he identifies a few ingredients all successful runners need. 'Intervals, distance days and rest days are all in there,'" he says. "I kind of cook the same way. You need your salt and your sugar and you know they all need to go in there, so you add them in, taste it and have a pretty good idea." Trail Runner Mag *online article by Alex Kurt, 8/23/14.*

Phase training (also known as periodization[1]) is a training technique that has worked well for me over the years. It was suggested while training with Dr. Cooper at Seattle Performance Medicine and personally tested over the years. The approach builds your mileage each week for three weeks followed by a recovery week. The building challenges your body and the rest week allows you to heal and absorb the workload. There is still a mileage goal, but I always tell my clients that rest is best, especially during recovery week. Rest weeks also give you a mental break, keeping you excited for the next block.

This plan is written on the assumption that people have time for long runs on the weekends and can make time for consistent training during the week. For your weekend runs, I would love to see you running terrain similar to your goal race. If you do not have access to similar racecourse terrain, play around with different locations on your long runs and vary your running routes. Look for a variety of options; one weekend could be hilly, the next flat. Explore long sustained climbs and descents versus rolling hills. Join different running groups to discover new locations as well as great training partners. The variety will help prepare your body and mind.

You will notice that I often put an easy run or short, steady run the day before a workout. I do this because I feel that the first day running after a day off feels a little wonky and out of tune. To me, it is best to do a workout the day after a comfortable run so that your system is ready to charge in the workout. I also put a short mellow run the day before a race for this same reason.

It is your responsibility to create a couple of core strength exercise routines that you will do. Always start with your biggest muscle groups, using a variety of exercises to build your strength. Do not feel limited by what I have written in the Core Strength Exercises Descriptions, EXTRA PIECES, page 215. I encourage you to try out the exercises and seek out additional, complementary exercises that aid in improving your running. Be creative on these days and do your best to feel like you made all of your muscles work. If you need guidance and more direction, I encourage you to hire a personal trainer or workout with friends.

---

1   Katch VL, McArdle WD, Katch FI. *Essentials of Exercise Physiology* (4th ed.) (2006). Baltimore, MD: Lippincott, Williams & Wilkins. p . 472-473.

I can spend as long as 45 minutes to an hour on core strength exercises, but also feel a sufficient workout after 30 minutes. As you become more confident with the movements, gravitate toward the more dynamic, engaging core strength exercises as opposed to single muscle group exercises—like bicep curls and tricep dips. Later, add weights for more resistance when you are confident you can maintain good form. Doing these workouts immediately after an easy run ensures your body will be limber. If you do not have time, it is great to make it a second workout of the day; be sure to warm up for 15–20 minutes. If you are tired after your run, it is best to separate the workouts so that you can recover in-between. Always be careful with your form. Practice good alignment and control as you move through the exercises.

A disclaimer to the strength program: The strength program I suggest and detail with exercise examples (Core Strength Descriptions, page 215) in this book are focused on building strength by enlisting stabilizing muscles, increasing flexibility (keeping muscles long and well aligned) and building muscle endurance (more explanation in Chapter Three: Tricks of the Trade, Core and Strength, page 25). I believe this focus alongside running helps prevent injury. When I am not training for a race, I find there is benefit to changing the focus of the strength program to build muscle mass and power. There are varying theories on what systems to train and when to train them relative to your race goals.

Stay engaged with your training plan. Make specific notes each day (See Athlete Log, EXTRA PIECES, page 214): how you felt, your running time and mileage, how you slept, what you ate, stress levels, etc. The more detailed you are, the more you will learn about your body. These notes are also helpful to review as you taper for your race as they will build confidence in your training. Try to repeat the series of workouts, sleep patterns and nutrition that led to positive energy and good outcomes. I hope to enable athletes to feel their bodies and to know when they should rest and when they should push. I would love to see everyone (non-runners too) tune in and become aware of exactly what their bodies need from movement, nutrition and sleep.

Good luck!

TOP TIPS

Throughout each of the training plans there are tips and quips to help motivate you. This page compiles the ones I feel are the most important into a list. This is your cheat sheet, a place to look when you need a little extra motivation or a reminder.

➜ Take care of the trails and the environment. I like to think of trails runners as stewards of the land because we connect with the special, beautiful places every time we head out the door.

➜ Take care of your body through your core strength exercises, foam rolling, stretching, eating, hydrating and sleeping. Tune in to the details of what helps you train and recover well as well as maintain a happy, healthy you!

➜ Use the Athlete Log (page 214) to track your mileage, exercise time, sleep and thoughts. The more information you track the better in-tune you will be with your body and your training.

➜ Fix the little issues before they become big issues.

➜ Connect with your local specialty run shop. In addition to helping you fit the best footwear and gear you will find amazing resources in the staff and a strong supportive community.

➜ Vary your training speed. You need speedy days as well as recovery pace days and everything in-between.

- → Volunteer at races. Learn what it is like to support other runners and what it takes to pull together a race. This knowledge will help you on race day to appreciate how much work is being put into the race you choose.

- → Trail work. Get out and build and help maintain your local trails. Some 100-mile events require trail work to run the race. I encourage everyone to sign up for a trail work party. It is a great way to build community, meet people and support the trail system that you train on.

- → Be grateful. You chose this and have the ability to do it.

- → Break up your long runs with different running buds. You may not be able to find someone to run 30 miles with you, but asking three or four to join you along the way will help pass the time, change up your pace and make for a fun outing.

- → Test your gear, your nutrition and all of your systems as frequently as possible. When you run your first ultra, the only thing that should be new to you is running the longest distance you've run to date.

- → Establish a relationship with a massage therapist and acupuncturist (if you like) and commit to regular bodywork. Investing the time and money to ensure your body stays healthy through your training is worthwhile.

- → You are your best teacher. Use this and other resources as your guides as you learn; tune in and listen to your body for the greatest lessons.

RUN WORKOUT DESCRIPTIONS

Run Workouts

When you warm up for any workout it is a good idea to include at least four strides. A great way to do a stride is on a marked football field (or imagine one). Start in the end zone and increase your pace over the first 10–30 yards. From 30 through 50 and to the other 30, you should be at a good sprint, use the remaining 30 yards to the other end zone to back off the pace and jog the final 10 yards. Catch your breath and turn around to repeat. Each direction is 1, so you only have to go down and back twice. Of course, adding a couple extra repeats is great if it makes you feel ready!

Additional Notes

If you want a technical method to figure out your heart rate zone (instead of going on feel and perceived effort) see Jason Karp M.S.'s article *Heart Rate Training for Improved Running Performance*—http://www.coachr.org/heart_rate_training_for_improved.htm.

Are you looking for a more scientific approach to finding your training pace? Consider playing with Dr. Jack Daniels VDOT calculator. http://runsmartproject.com/calculator/

THE CALENDAR SAYS

"X" miles easy.

Description

Think of this as a run where you spin out the legs. You want to feel comfortable breathing. A good test is if you can talk with someone while running or sing along if you are listening to music. On a scale of 1-10 this should feel like a 2 or 3.

Instructions

Try to execute the miles and feel good at the finish, like you could run more, but you are not going to. No matter the effort, it is always good to hydrate and think about necessary recovery nutrition afterwards.

THE CALENDAR SAYS
"X" miles steady.

Description
This is more of a focused run. Use the first mile to warm up and get into a good pace that you can maintain the remainder of the run. You should be able to talk, but will be a little winded as you do. 1–10, this should feel like a 5-6.

Instructions
You might be a little tired after these runs, but should not be as worked as you are following an interval or hill workout. No matter the effort, it is always good to hydrate and think about necessary recovery nutrition afterwards.

THE CALENDAR SAYS
Cardio.

Description
Elliptical machine, bike ride, rowing machine, swim. Running is cardio but I am using this note in your calendar for non-weight bearing activity, aka active recovery. 1–10, this is a 4–5.

Instructions
Do not feel limited to the times I have set. If you feel good, tack on 5–15+ minutes. If you are having a crummy day, cut it a little short.

Workout Example
40 minutes elliptical machine

OR

45 minutes hilly bike ride

OR

35 minutes swim laps

Additional Notes
You can also substitute cardio workouts on days that your body does not feel ready to run (Ex: day after workout, post race recovery). If you replace a steady run with a cardio workout, be sure to put in the appropriate effort to gain the desired training effect.

THE CALENDAR SAYS
Ladder.

Description
This is a build up of tempo effort runs. Warm up appropriately. When ready, increase speed to about 75–80 percent of max (this should feel like a 7–8 on the 1–10 scale) for the set amount of time and then recover for the same amount of time that you just ran. Example a "1, 2, 3" ladder is 1 minute up-tempo, 1 minute easy jog or walk, 2 minutes up-tempo, 2 minutes easy jog or walk, 3 minutes up-tempo, 3 minutes easy jog or walk. That is the workout. Then you cool down.

Instructions
I will write "1, 2, 3 ladder" or I could right "2, 4, 6 ladder." Adjust the up-tempos and recovery times. As you gain fitness I may write "half time recovery," which means you recover for only half of the time you just ran at tempo. Ex: "1, 2, 3 Ladder. Half-time recovery" = up-tempo 1 minute, recover 30 seconds, up-tempo 2 minutes, recover 1 minute, up-tempo 3 minutes, recover 90 seconds.

Workout Example
Ex: "2, 4, 6 LADDER"

THE CALENDAR SAYS
Pyramid.

Description
This is similar to a ladder workout, except after you climb the ladder you go back down as well. This is a longer workout!

Instructions
Example a "1, 2, 3, 2, 1 pyramid" is 1 minute up-tempo, 1 minute easy jog or walk, 2 minutes up tempo, 2 minutes easy jog or walk, 3 minutes up-tempo, 3 minutes easy jog or walk, 3 minutes up-tempo, 3 minutes easy jog or walk, 2 minutes up-tempo, 2 minutes easy jog or walk, 1 minute up-tempo, 1 minute easy jog or walk. That is the workout. Then you cool down.

Workout Example
Ex: "1, 2, 3, 2, 1 PYRAMID"

THE CALENDAR SAYS
5-minute repeats.

Description
This is my favorite workout for building endurance speed and it comes from coaching legend Dr. Jack Daniels. Warm up appropriately. You want to run the 5-minute intervals at 85–95 percent (Jack Daniels[1] says 97–100 percent[2]) of HRmax; about half marathon pace (10k pace if you are feeling awesome). The goal is to maintain the chosen pace for **all** intervals. It is important to find a challenging pace, but also one that you can maintain throughout the workout. This is a 8–9 on the 1–10 scale.

Instructions
If you can, run this workout on a track. With the measured 400-meter lap it is easy to break down the splits[3] to keep you on pace. 90 seconds per lap is 6 min/mile pace. The first couple will feel tough, but relatively easy compared to the remaining repeats. If you find you are falling off pace, then you probably started too fast. The short recovery window is what will challenge your system.

Workout Example
Ex: "4-6 x 5 min w/1 min recovery"

Additional Notes
Track etiquette: Give lane one to the fastest runner. Do not jog or cool down in lane one. Do not wear headphones on the track unless you can hear other runners.

THE CALENDAR SAYS
Hill workouts.

Description
Any of the above three workouts can be done on a sustainable graded hill.

Instructions
Warm up appropriately. Find a hill that is long enough and uninterrupted so you can run the allotted time. Jog downhill for your recovery windows.

Workout Example
Ex: "Ladder on Hill, 1, 2, 3, 4"

THE CALENDAR SAYS
Core strength exercises.

Description
Low weights and high reps. Pick the weights based on your ability to do three sets of 12–15 reps. Keep moving the entire time by working opposing muscle groups rather than resting between sets. Example: Do a set of bicep curls, then a set of tricep dips. Alternate back and forth with limited rest moving from one to the other. More example combinations include lat pull-downs and bench press. Focus on form and high reps. You are working on stability and endurance.

Instructions
I will write in "core strength exercises" two–three days a week. Exercises are described in detail in the Core Strength exercise descriptions (page xx). As you learn the exercises you may come up with your own routine. Definitely engage outside resources (friends, personal trainers, books, etc.) to find additional strengthening exercises to add to your routine. The key being that you are engaged and enjoy these workouts so that you will do them regularly.

Workout Example
Biceps 15 lbs 3x15, tricep dips 3x25, lat pull downs 70 lbs 3x12, bench press machine 45 lbs 3x12, one legged squats on BOSU bodyweight 3x25 each leg, crunches 3x50. (See core workout ideas p 215.)

THE CALENDAR SAYS
Rest.

Description:
Take the day easy; work on incorporating stretching on rest days and take care of any aches and pains from previous workouts. Active recovery is always good if your energy levels are high. If you are fatigued, take a full rest day, eat and hydrate well and get a good night's sleep.

1   Reference: Dr. Jack Daniels. (n.d.) Retrieved March 30, 2015. from Run Smart Project Website: http://runsmartproject.com/coaching/dr-jack-daniels/
2   Reference: Jack Daniels (Coach). (n.d.). Retrieved March 30, 2015 from Wikipedia: http://en.wikipedia.org/wiki/Jack_Daniels_(coach)
3   Reference: Calculator. (n.d.) Retrieved March 30, 2015 from Run Smart Project Website: http://runsmartproject.com/calculator/

COLOR CODE KEY

Rest and Easy days = green

Steady Effort and/or Long Distance days = blue

Speed/Hill (harder effort) days = yellow

If core strength exercises are added to the day = dotted border

FIRST 50K

Description: Recreational to consistent runner

Mileage: Average 20–30 miles/week

Race history: Occasional 5k or 10k, maybe one half-marathon

Previous longest training run: 10–13 miles

Minimum training time per week available: 6 hours/week

Training period: 6 months

Training Plan Notes

Before you start this program, promise me that you have been consistent with your mileage (at least 25 miles a week) for the last two–three months. Your body needs to have that consistency of training to ensure the strength in your muscles, ligaments and tendons to endure the next 24 weeks.

The hill and speed building phases are two weeks instead of three, and are introductions of these specific workouts. As we move into the endurance phase, you will continue to see both speed and hill workouts and sometimes both in the same week!

50K TRAINING PLAN

MONTHLY/WEEKLY OVERVIEW

If you prefer to train by time instead of miles, figure out your average minute/mile pace and multiply it by the scheduled miles. Ex1: 5 miles easy. Your easy pace is 10 minutes/mile. 5 x 10 = 50 minutes of easy running. Ex2: 8 miles steady. Your steady pace is 8:30. 8 x 8.5 = 68 minutes of steady running.

MONTH 1: TOTAL 79-92 MILES

Week 1 - Base Phase: 16–19 miles

Week 2 - Base Phase: 21–25 miles

Week 3 - Base Phase: 27–31 miles

Week 4 - Recovery: 15–17 miles

MONTH 2: TOTAL 111-129 MILES

Week 5 - Hills/Strength Phase: 29–31 miles

Week 6 - Hills/Strength Phase: 32–36 miles

Week 7 - Hills/Strength Phase: 35–45 miles

Week 8 - Recovery: 15–17 miles

MONTH 3: TOTAL 110-134 MILES

Week 9 - Speed Phase: 28–34 miles

Week 10 - Speed Phase: 31–37 miles

Week 11 - Speed Phase: 36–41 miles

Week 12 - Recovery: 15–22 miles

MONTH 4: TOTAL 145-168 MILES

Week 13 - Endurance Phase: 40–48 miles, long runs 6 and 12 miles

Week 14 - Endurance Phase: 44–50 miles, long runs 14 and 6 miles

Week 15 - Endurance Phase: 47–52 miles, long runs 15 and 8 miles

Week 16 - Recovery: 14–18 miles

MONTH 5: TOTAL 160-181 MILES

Week 17 - Endurance Phase: 45–52 miles, long runs 18 and 12 miles

Week 18 - Endurance Phase: 48–55 miles, long runs 20 and 8-10 miles

Week 19 - Endurance Phase: 53–56 miles, long runs 12 and 22 miles

Week 20 - Recovery: 14–18 miles

MONTH 6: TOTAL 153-172 MILES

Week 21 - Fine Tuning: 47–51 miles. Last back-to-back 20 and 10 miles

Week 22 - Fine Tuning: 39–43 miles. Last long run 18 miles

Week 23 - Taper: 25–33 miles

Week 24 - **50k RACE WEEK! Taper and rest up! 42–45 miles including race.**

Week 1

Base Phase / Total Miles: 16–19

This first week should be comfortable and familiar in relation to the training time you have been doing up to this point. We are building on the base that you bring to the program. Try to do every workout this week in the order they are presented so you can start the program committed to your calendar. There will be room for flexibility once you've established a connection with these workouts and consistency in your training. Keep track of your training using a running log (example page 214, Athletic Log).

MONDAY: 3 miles steady pace. Core strength exercises.	You want to feel good on this run. Perhaps it is a familiar neighborhood route or your favorite trail. It is a good idea to note your time. The runs you do this week are good benchmarks. Follow up with a core strength workout (see EXTRA PIECES: Core Workout Ideas, page 215). You can do this right after your run if you are feeling good. If core workouts have evaded you the last two–three months, be sure to start with bodyweight exercises and take the steps necessary to learn good form.
TUESDAY: 45 minutes cardio.	These cardio workouts are great active recovery as we move into the meat of this program. This week, the cardio workout (see Run Workout Descriptions, page 47 for cardio definition and effort level) helps you establish where (Local gym? Home fitness center?) you will do this non-weight bearing activity and keeps the body moving. Cardio examples: bike, elliptical, swim.
WEDNESDAY: Rest.	It might seem silly to build in a rest day so early in the program, but if you look ahead you will be thankful. These rest days (as well as the recovery weeks) are not only to rest your body; they are to give your mind a break. Finding the mental recharge in a rest day will increase your longevity through this program as well as in your running life.
THURSDAY: 5 miles steady. Core strength exercises.	You have two workouts today. Like Monday you can follow the run with the core strength exercises, or do one in the morning and one later in the day. If you split them up, use the downtime to hydrate and fuel well so your second workout feels just as strong. Keep in mind that if you do a lot of leg strengthening exercises you might feel tired for the run. I typically do the core strength exercises workout (see EXTRA PIECES: Core Workout Ideas, page 215) as the second workout of the day.
FRIDAY: 3 miles easy.	Active recovery the day after your double workout. Tomorrow is your long run, so really use these easy miles to flush out your legs so they feel good for tomorrow.
SATURDAY: 5–8 miles.	As your long run of the week and since it is on the weekend (hopefully you have a bit more time), use this opportunity to explore a bit. Find a new route or trail system that might have potential later in the program. Scope out larger trail networks so that you can get excited about the potential.
SUNDAY: Rest.	I am guessing that if you have been running 25 miles average a week a second rest day after a longer run will be a nice finish to the week. If you MUST move, you could do 30 minutes of cardio at an easy, flush-out-the-legs effort.

Week 2
Base Phase / Total Miles: 21–25

We have increased your miles this week a bit more than you will see in most training plans. You are able to do this because your weekly average leading in to the program was (should have been) at this mileage. If you are too tired, sore or quickly losing motivation, consider staying on the lower end of the weekly mileage to build your base. Please be aware of your body and its needs and do not push too hard too soon.

MONDAY: 3–4 miles steady pace. Core strength exercises.	If your schedule allows, break these into two separate workouts today. See if you prefer allowing the recovery in between to have a better second workout or if you prefer to lump the two together. Run in the morning and do a good core strength exercise workout in the afternoon.
TUESDAY: 45–50 min cardio.	Make sure your heart rate is in the steady zone (see page 48 for steady definition). You want to breathe harder and sweat during this cardio workout (unless you are in the pool—sweat is impossible to measure there). You shouldn't be able to read a book on the elliptical (unless you are really experienced) while working out. Focus on getting a good exertion out of this.
WEDNESDAY: 3 miles easy.	A few more easy miles this week and one less rest day compared to last week.
THURSDAY: 5 miles steady. Core strength exercises.	What worked for you last week? Did you split up the workouts? Did you follow the run with the core strength exercise workout? How about compared to Monday? Be sure to pick some different exercises and muscle groups than you focused on earlier this week.
FRIDAY: 4 miles easy.	Gauge how you are feeling after yesterday's run and know that you are running long tomorrow.
SATURDAY: 6–9 miles.	Did you find a place you loved last week? Do you want to explore it more? Or maybe it was a little disappointing. There is still time to find some amazing training grounds for your weekly (soon to be more) long run(s).
SUNDAY: Rest.	Enjoy! Foam rolling and stretching (see EXTRA PIECES, Recovery Movements, page 230) are amazing ways to make something of your rest days. A gentle yoga class (if you are into that) also fits in well here.

Week 3
Base Phase / Total Miles: 27–31

Look forward to your first workout on Friday this week! It really is something to enjoy. It might be the hardest thing you do all week and you will reap the most reward for the short time it will take you to do it.

MONDAY: 4 miles easy.	An easy morning run is always a good way to start the week.
TUESDAY: 5 miles steady pace. Core strength exercises.	Option: You can switch core strength exercises to Wednesday if it works better with your schedule.
WEDNESDAY: 50 min cardio.	Cardio does not mean lazy. Get the most out of this time. Push the resistance or incline grade up so that you have to work to keep moving.
THURSDAY: Rest.	Looking ahead, you have three solid days of running. Use this rest day to prepare.
FRIDAY: 15 min warm up. 1, 2, 3, 2, 1 PYRAMID (page 48) with equal recovery. 15 min cool down. ~5-7 miles total.	Here it is! Make sure you have an uninterrupted place to run, especially for the intervals. It is a good idea to stick to less technical terrain this first week, so that you can get a feel for the workout without having to do any fancy footwork.
SATURDAY: 5 miles easy. Core strength exercises.	The run will be a good follow up to your first workout. See these miles as a way to flush out your legs. Be careful on the core strength exercises after a day of speed (this is a tip that will be more relevant in the future). Sometimes speed work can make the muscles a little edgy. You do not want to cause an injury by lifting too much or moving awkwardly.
SUNDAY: 8–10 mile long run.	Now we are talking! It is exciting to me when the daily mileage hits the double digits. Do not go too crazy this early, and know that you've got some great long runs ahead of you.

Week 4
Recovery / Total miles 15–17

Your motto for this week is "Rest is Best." Active recovery and daily runs will keep the consistency in your body and running awareness as a part of your life. If you are struggling to get out the door due to lack of motivation, this is the week to back off from "pushing through." There are workouts and long runs for which you will need the extra mojo in the future. This week is not the one to use up that important psyche.

MONDAY: 3 miles easy or 40 min cardio.	
TUESDAY: 2–3 miles easy, Core strength exercises.	It is okay to bump up the effort/weight/reps/sets on the core strength exercises workouts this week if you are feeling good about where you are at recovery wise. With the extra time, since you are not running as much this week, and less workload from running, your body can recover from the extra output. As always, use good form, work the whole body and emphasize leg exercises one of the days.
WEDNESDAY: Rest.	
THURSDAY: 5 miles easy.	The running miles this week are to keep you consistent. If you feel the need to run a few more or a few less, just be sure to check in with your body and be aware of your recovery.
FRIDAY: No run. Core strength exercises.	
SATURDAY: 5–6 miles easy.	This is typically your long run day, but stick to the recovery week. It will pay off!
SUNDAY: Rest.	

Week 5
Hills/Strength Phase / Total Miles: 29–31

Moving into the hill workouts! This hill phase is three weeks with one week of recovery. Make the most of it! Learn the workouts and find landscapes that will work so you can accomplish this. These workouts will appear again in the endurance phase, so you will see them again.

MONDAY: 5 miles steady. Core strength exercises.	You've got this one down by this point.
TUESDAY: 3 miles easy.	Tomorrow will be tough. Be sure this run gets you fired up!
WEDNESDAY: 15 min warm up. HILL Workout: 2, 4, 2, 4, 2 with equal recovery. 15 min cool down. ~6-8 miles total.	Find a hill with a grade that you can run at a steady effort. Remember to keep your race in mind when deciding. Will the hill you choose benefit your training for your race? The intervals should be a little harder than your typical steady run effort. Recovery jog downhill in-between the efforts.
THURSDAY: Rest/active recovery. 20+ min cardio.	If you choose to do cardio, I think the movement will be good to help flush out yesterday's workout.
FRIDAY: 2 miles easy. Core strength exercises.	Continued recovery from that hill workout. Are you still feeling it in your legs?
SATURDAY: 8-mile long run of the week.	You will start to see back-to-back mileage over the weekends. As we move forward, these runs will be longer. I use back-to-back running to get your body used to running on tired legs (see Tricks of the Trade, Time on Feet, page 30). It is helpful to mimic your race course terrain on your weekend trail runs.
SUNDAY: 5 mile run, as you feel.	This can be at an easy or steady effort depending on how you are feeling at the end of the week.

Week 6
Hills/Strength Phase / Total Miles: 32-36

Not only are you incorporating hill workouts, your mileage in now climbing out of your base range comfort zone. Tune into your body and how it responds to the increasing workload. Are you more tired? How is your appetite? Be sure to feed these cues. Your body will tell you what it needs to continue training and increasing the stress. Note: If you are more tired, get more sleep. Caffeine will not help your body adapt as much as a 15-20 minute nap or an extra hour at night.

MONDAY: Rest.	If you can, do not think about running AT ALL today. I will not say this often, but I think it is good to take a mental break.
TUESDAY: 5-6 miles steady. Core strength exercises.	
WEDNESDAY: 4 miles easy.	To ready yourself for tomorrow's workout, throw a few 30-second surges into the later half of your run. Three to four will feel good (recover at your easy pace in-between) and leave you ready for a hard effort tomorrow.
THURSDAY: 15 min warm up. PYRAMID HILL Workout: 2, 4, 6, 4, 2 with equal recovery. 15 min cool down. ~7-9 miles.	You've done the pyramid workout before, but now you must use the interval minutes on a runnable incline. This is similar to last week's workout, except the middle effort is longer—the top of the pyramid. Your recovery time is equal to the interval time, which should feel sufficient to fully recover before starting the next push. Be sure to keep moving during recovery and mentally ready yourself to power uphill for each. Repeat.
FRIDAY: Rest/active recovery. You could squeeze in a second core strength exercise workout today!	If you opt for the core strength exercise workout, there is no doubt you will feel yesterday's hills. Keep this in mind and choose exercises that focus less on the legs and instead incorporate the whole body.
SATURDAY: 10-mile long run.	Another back-to-back mileage weekend. Be sure to hydrate, fuel and rest well in between so that you can have a good run tomorrow, too!
SUNDAY: 7-mile long run.	This might feel like a tough effort after yesterday and your solid week of training. If you need to back this down to an easy effort, that is okay. Still aim to cover the miles.

Week 7

Hills/Strength Phase / Total Miles: 35–45

The last two weeks I've had you on a runnable hill grade to get you used to the effort of hill running. Moving forward, the responsibility falls on you to be honest with yourself. What kind of course are you training for? Look at the elevation profile and try to mimic your hill workouts to best prepare you for your race. It is not going to do you any good to run on 5 percent grade when most of the hills in your race are 15 percent grade, in which case you should be training your power-hiking skills. And the opposite stands true as well. Power hiking steep grades will not better prepare you for rolling hills.

MONDAY: 4–6 miles easy. Core strength exercises.	You can switch today with Tuesday.
TUESDAY: Rest.	Recovery from your weekend. Some movement would be good today in preparation for tomorrow's workout.
WEDNESDAY: 15 min warm up. LADDER HILL Workout: 8, 6, 5, 4, 2 with equal recovery. 15 min cool down. ~8–12 miles.	You are climbing down the ladder in terms of time, but each of these intervals should be on a hill representative of your racecourse. If you are on a super steep grade and are power hiking, be sure that your heart rate is as high as it was on your runnable grade hill repeats last week. (See chapter three Tricks of the Trade, Power Hiking, page 27). If you think you want to use poles for your race, these hill repeats days are a good place to test them out. (See Trekking Poles, Gear page 185)
THURSDAY: 5 miles easy.	The miles continue through the rest of the week, but you have a recovery week to look forward to starting Monday. See if you can stick to the schedule and make this a strong training week for yourself!
FRIDAY: 3 miles steady. Core strength exercises.	Be sure these short miles are steady effort ones and not easy ones.
SATURDAY: 10–12 mile long run.	Wrap up this building phase with two solid runs this weekend. Go into your recovery week feeling like you earned it! Remember to choose a route that will help you prepare for your racecourse.
SUNDAY: 5–7 mile long run.	

Week 8
Recovery / Total Miles: 15–17

You've definitely earned this one! Hopefully you feel ready to chill a bit looking at the week ahead. Take note of how you are feeling each day. Are you tired early in the week? Does that improve by Wednesday or Thursday? How about your appetite? You may be super hungry even by mid-week. Your body could be making up for the potential caloric deficit incurred last week. Sleep and calorie needs will continue to increase as you get into longer training miles. It is good to pay attention now so that you are aware later.

MONDAY: Rest.	
TUESDAY: 2–3 miles easy. Core strength exercises.	Remember: It is okay to bump up the effort/weight/reps/sets on the core strength exercises during a recovery week if you are feeling good. With the extra time and less workload from running, your body can recover from the extra output. As always, use good form.
WEDNESDAY: 3 miles easy or 40 min cardio.	
THURSDAY: 5 miles easy.	
FRIDAY: No run. Core strength exercises.	Earlier in the week you may not have felt the extra energy for a tougher core strength exercises workout. How about today?
SATURDAY: 5–6 miles easy.	
SUNDAY: Rest.	

Week 9
Speed Phase / Total Miles: 28–34

If your training is anything like mine, the time is flying by! It is awesome to follow a calendar and check off the weeks, but it certainly seems to speed up time. As you roll into the speed phase it is a good time to check in with yourself. Are you getting what you want out of the workouts? Do the weeks feel like they are building in a manageable fashion? Are you resting when you are supposed to and pushing enough when the workouts demand? Tune in to your body to find the answers and adjust the workouts to help you achieve your mileage goals. If you are too tired and this feels impossible, repeat this first building block before moving on to more mileage. If you feel this is not enough, run on the upper end of the suggested mileage and enhance your core strength workouts with more exercises, repetitions and/or weight to build a solid foundation for the increasing mileage.

MONDAY: 4-6 miles easy.	
TUESDAY: 50 min cardio.	The harder work comes later in the week, so make sure you make the most of this depending on what your body needs (an extra push to sweat and breathe hard, or more of a spin out to flush the legs) and recover from it well through good hydration and well-timed nutrition.
WEDNESDAY: 5 miles steady. Core strength exercises.	These miles are to warm you up for tomorrow's workout. Consider saving more of the leg exercises (squats, lunges, etc.) for Friday, so that you have a bit more spring in your legs for tomorrow's ladder.
THURSDAY: 15 min warm up. 1, 2, 3, 4, 5 LADDER with equal recovery. 15 min cool down. ~6-9 miles.	You are climbing up the ladder. The intervals get longer as you go. Try to run the same pace for the 1-minute interval as you will for the 5-minute interval. (see Run Workout Descriptions, page 47) Really use the recovery time to bring your heart rate and breathing back under control. Continue moving at your easy pace, do not stop or walk. The active recovery is an important part of this workout.
FRIDAY: 3-4 miles steady pace. Core strength exercises.	Flush out the legs. Check in with how you are feeling after yesterday's effort. Take note if your legs are feeling a little off (tired, sore, stiff, achy), and be careful with movements while doing core strength exercises.
SATURDAY: Rest.	This is to encourage continued recovery from the ladder workout and to ready you for tomorrow's long run. If it would be better for your schedule to run long today and rest tomorrow, it is okay to make the switch.
SUNDAY: 10-mile long run.	Perhaps finding a running group will add some variety to this weekend's long run. If you are not interested in a running group, then look for a running partner that will push your pace a bit. If you prefer the solo time, try music. Unless you are adamantly against wearing ear buds, I find plugging in can encourage your pace on a long run. I typically do not run with music, but every once in a while it is a fun addition. If you do run with music, be aware of your surroundings, especially if you are in a high usage area. In that case, I recommend wearing only one ear bud so you can tune in to your surroundings as well as your tunes.

Week 10
Speed Phase / Total Miles: 31–37

During this phase, your weekly workout focuses on speed and leg turnover. Having worked on hills you have earned some strength. Now with these speed workouts, we still want to achieve those hard outputs. The effort will come more from within, rather than pushing against the terrain. The goal is setting a pace that is sustainable throughout the workout, while still pushing your edge. It may take a few attempts to figure out your ideal pace. I think you will get a feel for the effort based on your hill workouts. Reaching your goal times will come with practice.

Day	Workout	Notes
MONDAY: 5 miles steady. Core strength exercises.		Start the week right—there is some fun stuff to look forward to!
TUESDAY: 3 miles easy.		To ready yourself for tomorrow's workout, throw a few 30-second surges into the later half of your workout. Three to four will feel good (recover at your easy pace in between) and leave you ready for a hard effort tomorrow.
WEDNESDAY: 15 min warm up. PYRAMID Workout: 2, 4, 6, 4, 2 with equal recovery. 15 min cool down. ~6-9 miles.		This can be done on a track, treadmill, bike path or a mellow grade dirt road. Try to find a place that is easy/mellow footing and has minimal interruptions.
THURSDAY: Rest/active recovery. 20 min cardio.		Flushing out the legs the day after a workout is always a good idea.
FRIDAY: 2-4 miles easy. Core strength exercises.		Use these miles as continued recovery from your speed workout. Are you still feeling it in your legs? They might bounce back faster than the hill workouts.
SATURDAY: 10 miles.		Long run of the week.
SUNDAY: 5-7 mile run.		Back up yesterday's long run with another few miles today to top off your weekly mileage.

Week 11
Speed Phase / Total Miles: 36–41

This is a pretty solid mileage week and includes a tough speed workout on hump day. Learn to love the 5-minute repeat workout; it is a super beneficial one for pacing and training your threshold. It is hard and it hurts sometimes, but in the 60–90 minutes that it takes you to complete it, you will feel like you got more out of the time than a 3–4 hour run. And... recovery comes next week so you can totally do this.

MONDAY: Rest.	Stretching and foam rolling will be helpful! You can add some core strength exercises today, nothing too intense.
TUESDAY: 5 miles easy.	Use these miles to get your legs back under you for tomorrow's speed workout.
WEDNESDAY: 15–20 min warm up. 5 x 5 min (see Run Descriptions page 47) with 1 min recovery. 15 min cool down. ~8-11 miles.	You will see this workout throughout the rest of the training plan and it may take a couple of tries to figure out your pace. I find it super helpful to do this workout on a track. I can break down my pace and check in on my splits every 200 meters. If you have a local track, you may even find a few people interested in joining you. The best part is that everyone can run their own pace while simultaneously doing the workout together.
THURSDAY: 3-5 miles easy. Core strength exercises.	Definitely move today. These miles might feel a little funny, or you might feel super speedy. Be sure to keep them easy and flush out yesterday's workout.
FRIDAY: Rest.	
SATURDAY: 12-mile long run.	Perhaps this is the first time you've run this far. I think that is pretty cool! Venturing into your longest run distance is always an exciting step. Take the lessons you've learned from earlier long runs and stretch them out over the full distance.
SUNDAY: 8-mile long run.	You can do it! The legs might be a little tired and/or stiff from yesterday's effort. Take your time to warm up, fuel, hydrate and move through these fun miles. You are moving into a recovery week!

Week 12
Recovery / Total Miles: 15–22

Take note this week! For starters, acknowledge that this is the mid-way point of this training program. I encourage you to look ahead and see that the remainder of the plan is building, and fast. These first 11 weeks introduced you to some workouts and you should now be super dialed in on a core strength exercise routine that works for you. You have a solid base of miles and your body is tuned to receive the coming weeks of training. So take a breather this week. Get life in order to be able to accommodate the longer training hours that will be a significant part of the next three months. Build up that mojo and get excited! There is a lot of exploring, both on the trails and within yourself, to come.

MONDAY: Rest.	If you can, do not think about running AT ALL today. Take a mental break.
TUESDAY: 2–3 miles easy. Core strength exercises.	
WEDNESDAY: 3–5 miles easy or 45–60 min cardio.	Do one of these today and the other tomorrow.
THURSDAY: 3–5 miles easy or 45–60 min cardio.	Do the opposite of what you did yesterday.
FRIDAY: 2–3 miles. Core strength exercises.	
SATURDAY: 5–6 miles easy.	
SUNDAY: 3-5 miles as you feel.	

Week 13

Endurance Phase / Total Miles: 40–48. Long runs 6 and 12 miles.

The endurance phase will be tough. It should be! You've signed up to run your first ultra. You want to be ready. Focus on your consistency to prepare your body daily. Some weeks you will see both speed and hill workouts scheduled. Having multiple workouts in a week means that you need to spend just as much time managing your body and tending to aches and small pains before they cause problems. Foam rolling, stretching (see Recovery Movements, EXTRA PIECES, page 230) and of course your core strength exercises are huge factors in keeping your body healthy as you build these miles.

MONDAY: 5 miles steady. Core strength exercises.	Now you have played around with core strength exercises and know how to get a full body workout. Make sure to keep doing the exercises you don't really like and piece together workouts that increase overall strength.
TUESDAY: 15 min warm up. LADDER 1, 2, 3, 4, 5 with equal recovery. 15–20 min cool down. ~7–10 miles.	This is your speed workout of the week. Mellow terrain is best so that you work on turnover. Make these intervals a little quicker than normal, especially the 1 & 2 minute ones. You are climbing the ladder and then you are done and there is a lot of recovery in between each. Run smart and use good form!
WEDNESDAY: Rest from running. Core strength exercises.	Pay attention to your legs after the speed session yesterday. It is good to get in 45 minutes–1 hour on this workout today and hit the whole body. Just be careful not to tweak or aggravate anything that might be tender from your pace yesterday.
THURSDAY: 3–5 miles easy.	Keep in mind you have a tough workout tomorrow!
FRIDAY: 15–20 min warm up. PYRAMID HILL workout: 2, 4, 6, 4, 2 with equal recovery. 15 min cool down. ~7–10 miles.	Hopefully you have your legs back under you and are ready for this one. Find a runnable grade that gets your attention for this one. Find a place where you can run without interruptions. This is at your typical interval effort, breathing hard, difficult to speak, good form. Make it happen!
SATURDAY: 6 miles. (Warm up 2 miles, run steady 3 miles, cool down last mile.)	This should feel good after yesterday's hard effort. The middle 3 miles at a steady pace are to keep you honest.
SUNDAY: 12–mile long run.	Okay. You might be tired. It's been a tough week. You've got a day off from running tomorrow (don't forget core strength exercises though!). Do not do anything that is going to injure you. When you start a run fatigued, it is good to use these miles for mental training. Focus on managing your mind and body in a positive way. Utilize hydration and nutrition as aids to get you through this tired feeling. Taking in a few more calories than you are used to might make this a little easier. Definitely recover well afterward.

Week 14

Endurance Phase / Total Miles: 44–50. Long runs 14 and 6 miles.

The 5-minute repeats workout is back this week! Love to hate it, hate to love it. It is awesome and will do wonders as you recover from it. Your Saturday long run should be hilly, so think ahead about location and possible travel time if necessary.

MONDAY: Rest from running. Core strength exercises.	Core strength exercises are your only workout today. I hope it is a good one for you! If you feel like you need a complete rest day, then take today off and move the core strength exercise workout to tomorrow in addition to the miles. Sometimes a full rest day can do wonders.
TUESDAY: 5-6 miles easy.	
WEDNESDAY: 15 min warm up. 5–6 x 5 min with 1 min recovery. 15-20 min cool down. ~8-11 miles.	
THURSDAY: 8 miles steady.	This might be a little tough after yesterday's workout.
FRIDAY: 3–5 miles easy. Core strength exercises.	
SATURDAY: 14-mile long run.	You do not have a hill workout this week, so make this run a hilly one! Similar to your racecourse if possible. You should work the hills by pushing the pace. Think about how you want to feel and perform in your race while running or power hiking uphill.
SUNDAY: 6-mile run.	Don't slack on these; run strong. This is your back-to-back. It's short, but you want these miles to feel like miles 20–26 of your 50k.

Week 15

Endurance Phase / Total Miles: 47–52. Long runs 15 and 8 miles.

Your mileage has been steady for a while and this is the last week of your first endurance building phase. Look forward to next week's recovery! We are getting into your biggest weekly mileage, which means a lot of things: More time on your feet, more energy output, bigger appetite and extra sleep to recover properly. Budget your time wisely and prepare meals and gear bags ahead of time to save you time and ensure good recovery fuel and hydration.

MONDAY: Rest.	Finally a full rest day!
TUESDAY: 9-mile run. Warm up for the first 2–3. Keep the middle 3 steady. Cool down the last 3.	This is a big run for your first run of the week. Really warm up and cool down at a comfortable pace. Push the middle 3–4 miles so that you feel your effort (Tempo pace). These middle miles are your speed miles this week.
WEDNESDAY: 5 miles steady. Core strength exercises.	You have core strength exercises on either side of your hill workout this week, so think about which day makes the most sense to put some emphasis on your legs, or if you want to just go for full body both days.
THURSDAY: 15–20 min warm up. HILL Workout: 3 x 5 min with 3 min recovery. 3 x 2 min with 1 min recovery. 15 min cool down.~7-10 miles.	This workout is similar to the 5-minute repeats you've done, but now you will do them on a hill and with a bit more recovery in between. For the second set of 3 x 2 minutes, try to pick up the pace compared to what you were doing the 5-minute intervals.
FRIDAY: 3–5 miles easy. Core strength exercises.	
SATURDAY: 15-mile long run.	Try to keep the middle 5–8 miles at a good up-tempo pace! Hills never hurt to add and will make you tougher.
SUNDAY: 8-mile run.	You have a full rest day tomorrow and you are going into a recovery week! Make these miles count.

Week 16
Recovery / Total Miles: 14–18

This recovery week should be well timed. If your weekly mileage coming into this program was around 30 miles per week, you now have been running more than that for over the past two phases. REST UP! Let all of that work absorb into your body. Continue to fuel and hydrate appropriately so your body can heal from the training and get stronger. You have one more endurance phase that you want to be ready for. This downtime is the preparation you need to charge again soon.

MONDAY: Rest.	Two full rest days this week. One to start the week and one to finish it off. If it feels like you need an additional rest day, either Wednesday or Thursday would be a good one to swap out. You can move the Wednesday or Thursday workout to Sunday.
TUESDAY: 3–4 miles easy. Core strength exercises.	
WEDNESDAY: 3–5 miles easy or 45–60 min cardio.	Do one of these today and the other tomorrow.
THURSDAY: 3–5 miles easy or 45–60 min cardio.	Do the opposite of what you did yesterday.
FRIDAY: 3 miles. Core strength exercises.	Hopefully you are feeling more recovered and strong. If so, this would be a good day to have a solid core strength exercise training session.
SATURDAY: 5–6 miles easy.	
SUNDAY: Rest.	If you can, do not think about running AT ALL today. Do not train physically or mentally today, just be.

Week 17
Endurance Phase / Total Miles: 45–52. Long runs 18 and 12 miles.

As your weekend back-to-back runs get longer and longer it is a good time to really start tuning in to the mental aspect of your training. Running ultras is very physical, and it is pretty straight-forward on how to train. It is the mental aspect that will see you through to the ultra finish line. How you perceive yourself, your training and your ability becomes more important as you lengthen the distance of your goals. Try some of the mental training tips in Train Your Brain starting on page 33 out on your long runs this weekend and in the coming weeks.

MONDAY: 3 miles easy. Core strength exercises.	These miles are really to warm you up for the speed workout tomorrow.
TUESDAY: 15 min warm up. (Like Ladder): 2, 4, 2, 4, 2, 4, 2 with half time recovery. 15 min cool down. ~6-9 miles.	You are not climbing ladder this week like before, but it is a speed/interval workout and should be executed similarly. This will be hard because I've cut your recovery time in half. The intervals are not super long, but you will start to feel the lack of recovery time toward the final repeats.
WEDNESDAY: 6-mile steady run.	Flush out yesterday's workout.
THURSDAY: 2-4 miles easy. Core strength exercises.	Get ready for some BIG miles this weekend.
FRIDAY: Rest.	There is not a hill workout this week, but I highly recommend planning the weekend to mimic your racecourse. If there are hills, make one or both of your weekend runs match the racecourse profile the best you can.
SATURDAY: 18-mile long run.	These are two significant distance back-to-back weekend runs. Plan on these taking time, not only to run, but also to prepare gear, food and recovery eats, commute and recover.
SUNDAY: 10-12 mile long run.	Don't be surprised if all you want to do come Sunday afternoon (assuming you did your run in the morning) is take a nap. If you can get horizontal for even 20 minutes I highly encourage it. A 20-30 minute nap will do wonders for your recovery and help you finish the day with a smile.

Week 18
Endurance Phase / Total Miles: 48–55. Long runs 20 and 8–10 miles.

Week two of a three-week building phase can be mentally tough. You are in the thick of the mileage, that is, you already have a week's worth of miles built up and still have next week. This is where the mental training comes into play. You can and should use the mental training techniques to work through these tougher miles. You will train your mind for the tough times that could show up during your race. Be kind to yourself, but also test your edge and learn what you are made of. If your calendar will not allow the time required for the weekend long runs (perhaps you have flexibility during the week), check out the alternate weeks for weeks 18 and 19. These should give you some ideas on how to log your miles early and free up your weekends.

MONDAY: 4 miles easy. Core strength exercises.	
TUESDAY: 15 min warm up. 6 x 5 min with 1 min recovery. 15 min cool down. ~7-10 miles.	Remember this one? It is here to stay (other than your recovery and taper weeks).
WEDNESDAY: Rest.	
THURSDAY: 7 miles steady.	Work some rolling hills into your route and push the pace a bit on the ascents.
FRIDAY: 2-4 miles easy. Core strength exercises.	Gauge how you are feeling after yesterday's run and know that you are running long tomorrow. Think about giving yourself as much recovery time as possible. Hint: Do both of these workouts in the morning so you have the remainder of the day to hydrate, fuel, rest and prep for tomorrow.
SATURDAY: 20-mile long run.	Use these weekend long runs to prepare yourself for the race. Running on similar terrain is awesome! Also think about testing all of your gear before the race. All clothing. All nutrition. Have everything dialed!!
SUNDAY: 8-10 mile long run.	

Week 18 Alternate

Endurance Phase / Total Miles: 48–45. Long runs 20 and 8–10 miles.

Use this schedule if weekend long runs do not fit into your schedule. This alternate to week 18 will hold your attention mid-week. It can be difficult to work in these longer runs in addition to your normal weekly commitments. Plan accordingly and remember the weekend (you are trying to open up) is right around the corner!

MONDAY:
4 miles easy.
Core strength exercises.

TUESDAY:
15 min warm up. 6 x 5 min with 1 min recovery. 15 min cool down.
~7-10 miles.

WEDNESDAY:
7 miles steady.

THURSDAY:
12-mile AM run and 8-mile PM run OR 20-mile long run.

If you have a typical workday, you can split your long run in to two runs. If you have a day off mid-week, do the longest of your two runs on the day off and split up the second day's mileage into two. Ideally you will complete some of these long runs in one push so that you can get used to time on your feet. If your schedule does not allow the block of time required, running twice in one day to achieve the mileage is a good alternative.

FRIDAY:
8-10 mile long run.

This makes for a tough week for sure! Tuesday through Friday are all solid days. It is doable with the training that you have. You need to make sure you are getting the sleep and nutrition to recover in-between all of these.

SATURDAY:
2-4 miles easy.
Core strength exercises.

SUNDAY:
Rest.

Week 19

Endurance Phase / Total Miles: 53–56. Long runs 12 and 22 miles.

The bulk of this week comes over the weekend. Early in the week, do some of the mental preparation techniques that will steer you away from wasting energy and will psyche you up for your long miles. This is good mental strategy practice for your taper weeks (23 and 24) leading in to the race. It will be helpful to clear your calendar from too many extra activities. You should be focused on eating, sleeping and running. There will be some down time, of course, but it might be your best plan to focus on your training runs and not overbook yourself otherwise.

MONDAY: Rest.	
TUESDAY: 5 miles easy. Core strength exercises.	Pay attention to your recovery from the weekend long runs. Wednesday's workout is tough. Take these miles and the core strength exercises workout easy if you need more recovery before tomorrow.
WEDNESDAY: 15 min warm up. 7–8 x 5 min with 1 min recovery. 15 min cool down. ~9-12 miles.	This will definitely be a tough one. 7 and 8 repeats of the 5 minutes repeats (see Run Workout Descriptions, page 47) is always tough for me. I know people that do upwards of 10-12 repeats, but 8 seems to be a worthy workout. If you do the math, this is 40 minutes at a much faster than ultra race pace effort. (10 would be 50 minutes and 12 an hour). As race distances increase and finishing times are more competitive, the training bar raises. The most important thing you can do is hold your pace for all of the repeats and feel good after the workout. You have your longest block of mileage this week, so you definitely want to do this workout no later than Wednesday, so that you have the next two days to recover.
THURSDAY: Rest or 30-40 minute cardio.	You can add some core strength exercises if you are feeling it.
FRIDAY: 5 miles steady.	Pack your kit for tomorrow's run. Plan out a few food options that you are thinking you would like to eat during the race and try them out on these next two training runs. Start to think about the clothing you would like to wear in your race and use these pieces. It is best to dial in as much as possible prior to your race so that the only "new" experience is going your farthest distance to date.
SATURDAY: 22-mile long run.	This is your longest mileage on a back-to-back weekend. Be sure to take really good care. This is the weekend to focus on running, eating and sleeping. Minimize extra work and social activities.
SUNDAY: 12-mile long run.	

Week 19 Alternate
Endurance Phase / Total Miles: 51–56. Long runs 22 and 12 miles.

This is the alternate for week 19, in the case that you need your weekend open. This alternate makes for a tough Monday through Thursday. Be ready for consistent, solid days of running. Keep focused, take care of yourself and be sure to get lots of sleep and good nutrition.

MONDAY: Rest.	Use this rest day to prepare for your mid-week long runs. Pack your kit, plan out the food options you are thinking about using race weekend. Use the two long run days to test race day gear and food. It is best to dial in as much as possible prior to your race so that the only "new" experience is going your farthest distance to date.
TUESDAY: 5 miles easy. Core strength exercises.	Pay attention to your recovery from the weekend long runs. Wednesday's run is long and you follow it up with a tough workout on Saturday. Take these miles and the core strength exercises workout easy if you need more recovery before tomorrow.
WEDNESDAY: 12 mile AM run and 6–8 mile PM run OR 20–22-mile run.	This is your longest mileage in a back-to-back effort. Be sure to take really good care. This is the week to focus on running, eating and sleeping. Minimize extra work and social activties.
THURSDAY: 12-mile long run OR 8 miles AM & 4 miles PM.	
FRIDAY: Rest or 30–40 minutes cardio.	
SATURDAY: 15 min warm up. 7 x 5 min with 1 min recovery. 15 min cool down. ~9-12 miles.	If you took a rest day yesterday, you might need a little longer warm up to feel good and ready for this workout. Also, be kind to yourself, your normal 5-minute pace may not be achievable considering the mileage you have already done this week.
SUNDAY: 5 miles easy.	

Week 20
Recovery / Total Miles: 14–18

We are getting close now. Can you believe that this is your last recovery week before your race? Crazy to think! But don't get too worked up just yet. There are still a couple of weeks to fine tune your dialed machine and then your taper period will feel a lot like a long recovery week. The cool thing about your taper is that by now you have taught your body how to recover and absorb the training. You know how to recharge, your muscles bounce back so that you can perform better and stronger for the next phase, or in this case, the race. Keep this in mind as you recover this week, pay attention to how your body turns around from tired to recovered.

MONDAY: Rest.	This recovery week should feel pretty familiar by now. I hope it works for you. If there are some runs or workouts that you prefer during your recovery week, I definitely encourage you to do what feels good. Keep "Rest is Best" in mind this week.
TUESDAY: 3-4 miles easy. Core strength exercises.	
WEDNESDAY: 3-5 miles easy or 45-60 min cardio.	
THURSDAY: Rest.	
FRIDAY: 3 miles. Core strength exercises.	
SATURDAY: 5-6 miles easy.	
SUNDAY: Rest.	

Week 21

Fine Tuning / Total Miles: 47–51. Last back-to-back 20 and 10 miles.

Fine tuning is as it sounds. Fine tune you. Fine tune your gear. (Read Race Day Preparations: Ready? Set? page 199) You have learned a lot about your body up to this point, now apply this knowledge in these next two weeks. Do the workouts that give you the best feeling. Eat the foods and time your recovery so that you feel dialed before, during and after every run. Read through the course description, visualize and project your best race. Make your body work for you. Make your mind work for you.

MONDAY: Rest/active recovery. Core strength exercises.	
TUESDAY: 15 min warm up. 5-7 x 5 min with 1 min recovery. 15 min cool down. OR 15 min warm up. HILL workout: 1, 3, 5, 7, 3, 1 with half time recovery. 15 min cool down. ~7-11 miles.	You have an option today: speed or hills. Pick one. Do not do both. If you pick speed today, be sure to make Thursday's run hilly and work the hills a bit. If you pick hills today, be sure to run a speedier course and throw in a good tempo and a couple of surges.
WEDNESDAY: Rest/active recovery.	
THURSDAY: 7 miles steady.	Be sure to read the notes from Tuesday; make this a good workout-type run.
FRIDAY: 3 easy miles. Core strength exercises.	
SATURDAY: 20-mile long run.	Dial it in! This weekend is a great one to test any new gear you are thinking of using on race day. If you want to completely geek out, you could even practice an aid station run through with your crew (I can honestly say I've never actually practiced it, but I've definitely talked through different scenarios). All of the preparation will help you plan what to pack. Start making a list (or use the Race Packing List, EXTRA PIECES, page 226), and write down little things you might not remember later. It is best to jot down a list of what is in your pack while you are using it (or just after) rather than trying to think of what you use two days later.
SUNDAY: 10-mile long run.	

Week 22

Fine Tuning / Total Miles: 39–43. Last long run 18 miles.

This week is about dialing back the mileage, putting in some solid days when you run a workout or long run and to just keep moving the rest of the week. It is time to start feeling good, strong and ready. You do not have to be completely dialed yet, but you should feel your body working toward that final preparation.

MONDAY: 3 miles easy. Core strength exercises.	If 40 minutes of cardio sounds more appealing on either Monday or Wednesday, then that can be helpful active non-weight bearing movement.
TUESDAY: 15 min warm up. 6-8 x 5 min with 1 min recovery. 15 min cool down. OR 15 min warm up. HILL workout: 1, 3, 5, 7, 3, 1 with half time recovery. 15 min cool down. 8-12 miles.	Make the opposite choice from last week. If you opted for hills in week 21, shoot for 7–8 x 5-minute repeats this week. If you chose speed last week, do the hill workout. If you really have grown to love the 5-minute repeat workout, and you think it will serve you best for your race preparations, go for your best effort and do one more repeat than you did last week. This is your last hard workout before the race.
WEDNESDAY: 3 miles easy. Core strength exercises.	If you are really into the core strength exercises (I hope you are!) and enjoy putting time into getting stronger (sweet!) please make this your last hard core strength exercise workout. You have core strength exercises in the taper weeks, but those should be body weight exercises and nothing that will make you sore.
THURSDAY: Rest.	
FRIDAY: 7 miles hilly and steady.	
SATURDAY: 18-mile long run.	This is your last long run! Make this a GREAT one! Test all of your race gear and your nutrition plan. Feel awesome afterwards ... recover smart.
SUNDAY: Rest.	If you can, do not think about running AT ALL today.

Week 23

Taper / Total Miles: 25–33

This might feel like a long taper, but I think it will be worth it. You have put in some amazing miles leading up to this point and now it is time for your body to do what it has learned throughout this program: recover.

MONDAY: Rest/active recovery.	If you haven't already, now would be a great time to start dialing in your crew or drop bags. Whatever system you are going to use for the race, figure it out now. It is best to work on these things early, rather than too close to the race when other last minute worries ail you. Having this taken care of will ease your mind. I have included thoughts on crew preparations on page 173 and drop bags prep on page 178.
TUESDAY: 3–5 miles steady. Core strength exercises.	If 40 minutes of cardio sounds more appealing on either Tuesday or Thursday (or both!) then that can be helpful, active, non-weight bearing movement. Remember to keep your core strength exercise workouts effective, but do not overdo it.
WEDNESDAY: 15 min warm up. 4–5 x 5 min with 1 min recovery. 15 min cool down. ~6-8 miles.	This should feel easy and you should start to feel like you are going to be ready for the race weekend. This is a good time to check in on what you need to do to be rested and primed for the race weekend.
THURSDAY: 3–5 miles easy. Core strength exercises.	
FRIDAY: Rest.	
SATURDAY: 8–10 mile trail run.	Run within yourself. Have fun! Visualize what you are going to feel like next week at this time. You might try running this at the same time as the race starts (only if you can ensure a good night sleep on either side). It would be a good way to ready your system.
SUNDAY: 5 miles.	Take this as an easy spinout for your legs. This is just to keep you from starting the taper tantrums too early. If you feel like rest would be better, then go for it! A little active recovery or cardio is also a good option.

Week 24
50k RACE WEEK! Taper and rest up! 42–45 miles including race miles.

Are the taper tantrums setting in for you? Definitely read up on that distracting energy in chapter five, Train your Brain, Q&A, question #4, page 38. Keep calm and train your mind. The mental aspect is what is going to get you through. These final days before the race, when you are feeling antsy and would prefer to just be running, use the time to focus your mind and visualize a great run this weekend. The energy will be much better spent training your mind than wasting it on excess movement. Remember, there is no training run you can do this week that will make your race better. Only rest, sleep and good nutrition/hydration will give you the positive impacts you are looking for.

MONDAY: Rest … You can do some of your favorite core strength exercises, but don't do anything to make you sore or that you cannot recover from.	
TUESDAY: 10-minute warm up. 3-5 x 2 min with 1 min jog/recovery. 10 min cool down. ~5-6 miles.	This is just to make you feel good and fast. Remember, nothing you do this week will have time to settle in your body and make you have a better race. The runs this week are purely good movement and are scheduled to help keep you calm.
WEDNESDAY: 3-5 miles easy.	This can be a rest day or 30-40 minute cardio workout. Really listen to what will be best for you!
THURSDAY: Rest.	Train your mental. Period.
FRIDAY: 3 miles easy. 4 x 100m strides.	This is so that you sweat and work out some kinks the day before your race. Remember I feel it is best to move the day before you put out your best effort. You might feel slow and a little clunky after so much rest. Remember all of your visualization and be positive. Believe that this is working out the tiny hitches before you really go.
SATURDAY: 50k RACE	How exciting! Race day is here! Please read Chapter twelve, GO!, page 205 for my last little tidbits … I'm excited for you and more importantly, I hope you are excited for you.
SUNDAY: CELEBRATE!	

FIRST 50M OR 100K

Description: Consistent runner

Mileage: Average 38–50 miles/week

Race History*: Ran at least one marathon or a 50k

Previous longest training run: 22–25 miles

Minimum training time per week available: 10 hours/week

Other details: Has an understanding of incorporating hill workouts and speed workouts

Training period: 4–6 months

* This is the base, or minimum from which a runner should start the 50-mile or 100-km training program. If you have completed more marathons or 50ks, or your weekly mileage averages are higher, this is still a good place to start.

Training Plan Notes

Timing: The time required to train for this distance depends on whether you are piggybacking this race with a 50k (you will need 4 months) or starting from your base (6 months).

➜ If you are starting this program from a solid base averaging 40 miles/week, start from the beginning.

➜ If a 50k race is not in your recent past, consider running a 50k race at week 15. (See Alternate Week 15, Month 4.)

➜ If you recently ran a 50k and recovered for 2–4 weeks, start this plan at week 4 or week 8.

50-MILE TRAINING PLAN

MONTHY/WEEKLY OVERVIEW

If you prefer to train by time instead of miles, figure out your average minute/mile pace and multiply it by the scheduled miles. Ex1: 5 miles easy. Your easy pace is 10 minutes/mile. 5 x 10 = 50 minutes of easy running. Ex2: 8 miles steady. Your steady pace is 8:30. 8 x 8.5 = 68 minutes of steady running.

MONTH 1: TOTAL 121-138 MILES

Week 1 - Base Phase: 25–31 miles

Week 2 - Base Phase: 30–35 miles

Week 3 - Base Phase: 36–42 miles

Week 4 - Recovery (or Start) week: 30 miles

MONTH 2: TOTAL 146–176 MILES

Week 5 - Building (Speed) 37–45 miles, long runs 12–14 and 8–10 miles

Week 6 - Building (Speed) 44–48 miles, long runs 12–14 and 8 miles

Week 7 - Building (Speed) 38–50 miles, long runs 5–8 and 12–15 miles

Week 8 - Recovery 27–33 miles

MONTH 3: TOTAL 145–182 MILES

Week 9 - Building (Hills) 38–48 miles, long runs 10–12 and 7–9 miles

Week 10 - Building (Hills) 40–49 miles, long runs 12–14 and 10–12 miles

Week 11 - Building (Hills) 48–57 miles, long runs 18–20 and 14–16 miles

Week 12 - Recovery 19–28 miles

MONTH 4: TOTAL 182-219 MILES

Week 13 - Building (Endurance) 51–62 miles, long runs 8–10 and 18 miles

Week 14 - Building (Endurance) 55–65 miles, long runs 18–20 and 10–12 miles

Week 15 - Building (Endurance) 57–68 miles, long runs 20–22 and 9–11 miles

Week 16 - Recovery 19–24 miles

MONTH 4 ALTERNATE: TOTAL 194–227 MILES

Week 13 - Building (Endurance) 51–62 miles, long runs 8–10 and 18 miles

Week 14 - Building (Endurance) 55–65 miles, long runs 18–20 and 10–12 miles

Week 15 – 50k race + 38–45 miles = 69–76 miles, long runs 31 and 10–12 miles

Week 16 – Recovery 19–24 miles

MONTH 5: 228–259 MILES

Week 17 - Building (Endurance) 61–69 miles, long runs 25 and 14 miles

Week 18 - Building (Endurance) 64–75 miles, long runs 25–28 and 12–15 miles

Week 19 - Building (Endurance) 75–80 miles, long runs 28–30 and 15 miles

Week 20 - Recovery 28–35 miles

MONTH 6: 189–212 MILES

Week 21 - Fine Tuning: 62-66 miles, last back-to-back 25 and 12 miles, long runs 25 and 12 miles

Week 22 - Fine Tuning: 43–51 miles, last long run 18–22 miles

Week 23 - Taper: 24–32 miles

Week 24 - 50M RACE WEEK! Taper and rest up! 60–63 miles including race

Week 1
Base Phase / Total Miles: 25–31

This first week should be comfortable and familiar in relation to your current training and level of fitness. We are building on the base and consistency that you bring to the program. Try to do every workout this week in the order they are presented so that you start off committed to your calendar. There will be room for flexibility once you've established a connection with these workouts. Keep track of your training using a running log (example page 214, Athlete Log, EXTRA PIECES).

Day	Workout	Description
MONDAY:	Warm up 5–10 min. 3 miles steady pace. Cool down 5–10 min. Core strength exercises. ~5–7 miles.	Be sure to warm up (walk/jog) at a comfortable pace for 5–10 minutes. Then run 3 miles steady. Finally, cool down for 5–10 minutes. Follow your run with a core strength exercise workout. Your muscles will be warm and ready.
TUESDAY:	45 min cardio.	These cardio workouts (see Cardio Description in Run Workouts Descriptions, page 48) are great active recovery as we move into the meat of this program. This week, the cardio workout helps you establish where you will do this non-weight bearing activity (Local gym? Home fitness center?) and keeps the body moving. Ex: bike, elliptical, swim.
WEDNESDAY:	3–5 miles easy. Core strength exercises.	You have two workouts today. You can follow the run with the core strength exercise workout, or do one in the morning and one later in the day. If you split them up, use the downtime to hydrate and fuel well so your second workout feels just as strong. Keep in mind that if you do a lot of leg exercises you might feel tired for the run. I typically do the core strength exercise workout as the second workout of the day.
THURSDAY:	6 miles steady.	Use the first mile to warm up, run steady for 4–5 miles and cool down the final mile (~10 minutes).
FRIDAY:	Rest from running. Core strength exercises.	You can take this as a complete rest day if you feel you need it. This is the 3rd core strength exercise workout of the week, so see it as extra credit if you are feeling good.
SATURDAY:	5 miles easy.	
SUNDAY:	6–8 miles as you feel.	

Week 2

Base Phase / Total Miles: 30-35

Pay attention to your body, how your muscles and joints feel, your appetite and sleep requirements as you continue into these weeks. Write down notes associating what you did with how you feel, so that you can later reference and learn what works best for you.

MONDAY: 5 miles steady. Core strength exercises.	If your schedule allows, try breaking these two workouts up today. Run in the morning and do a good core strength exercise workout in the afternoon. See if you feel a difference in what you are able to get out of each workout compared to lumping them together.
TUESDAY: 45-50 min cardio.	Make sure you are getting your heart rate up. You want to work at the steady output level and sweat during this cardio workout (unless you are in the pool; sweating is impossible to measure there). You should not be able to read a book on the elliptical (unless you are really experienced) while working out. Focus on getting a good exertion out of this.
WEDNESDAY: 6 miles easy.	
THURSDAY: 3-5 miles easy. Core strength exercises.	What worked for you last week? Did you split up the workouts or follow the run with the core strength exercises? How about compared to this Monday? Be sure to pick some different exercises and muscle groups than you focused on earlier this week.
FRIDAY: Rest.	Enjoy! Foam rolling and stretching are amazing ways to make a little something of your rest days. A gentle yoga class (if you are into that) also fits in well here.
SATURDAY: 10-12 miles.	Did you find a trailhead that you love last week? Do you want to go explore it more? Or maybe it was a little disappointing. There is still time to find your amazing training grounds for your weekly (soon to be more) long run(s).
SUNDAY: 6-7 miles steady.	This is your first taste of a back-to-back longer distance runs (see Trick of the Trade, Time on Feet, page 30). Listen to your body. If holding your steady pace isn't working, don't worry just yet. Work on your effort level. You might not be running as fast (min/mile), but your heart rate will show your effort.

Week 3
Base Phase / Total Miles: 36–42

The miles are building quickly and you have your first workout this week! (See Run Workout Descriptions, Pyramid, page 48.) This week wraps up with bigger miles over the weekend and a back-to-back test sandwiched between two rest days.

MONDAY: 4–6 miles easy.	An easy morning run is always a good way to start the week and work out the kinks from your weekend back-to-back.
TUESDAY: 50 min cardio. Core strength exercises.	Cardio does not mean lazy. Get the most out of this time.
WEDNESDAY: 6 miles. (2 warm up, 2 steady, 2 cool down.)	The middle two steady miles are to prep your legs for the quicker turnover on tomorrow's workout. Do not get too excited and accidentally run too fast today. The workout is tomorrow and you want to feel good for it.
THURSDAY: 15 min warm up. 1, 2, 3, 4, 3, 2, 1 PYRAMID with equal recovery. 15 min cool down. ~6-8 miles.	Here it is! Make sure you have an uninterrupted place to run, especially for the intervals. It is a good idea to stick to mellow, less technical terrain this first week, so that you can get a feel for the workout without having to do any fancy footwork. This will take you a little over 1 hour to complete (15 min warmup + 20 min hard + 20 min recovery in between + 15 min cool down).
FRIDAY: Rest from running. Core strength exercises.	Take note of how your body feels after the speedier running yesterday. Be sure to warm up properly and be careful not to tweak anything while working on core strength exercises. Consider doing only body weight exercises and not adding weight. The core strength exercises are your only workout for the day; focus on hitting all the major muscle groups for a full body workout. This might require a little extra time.
SATURDAY: 12-mile long run.	
SUNDAY: 8-10 mile long run.	

Week 4
Recovery (or Start) Week / Total Miles: 30

This is your final week of the base phase. Some people love the recovery week. Others hate it because they do not get to train as much. Either way you will come to appreciate it as we build into longer and harder training weeks. The recovery weeks mark the end of each phase and allow your body the time necessary to absorb the work. While this first recovery week may seem a little early in the training plan, I think it is a good idea to give you a break in the action, recharge the batteries and prep you for the coming weeks.

If you are coming into this week as week 1 of your plan, shoot for 35–38 miles total for the week, adding in 5 on Monday and increasing the mileage on a couple of the shorter runs.

MONDAY: Rest.	You just finished three pretty solid weeks and this rest day kicks off your recovery week. Get in the habit of adding yoga, light stretching and foam rolling (see Recovery Movements, EXTRA PIECES, page 230) to your rest day.
TUESDAY: 50 min cardio.	This is active recovery and is a good way to spin out the legs. During your recovery week, you don't have to kill it (i.e., work at high intensity) on this workout, but you should build up a good sweat and feel stretched out and less creaky when you are done.
WEDNESDAY: 5 miles steady. Core strength exercises.	Take this core strength exercise workout as an opportunity to try a few new exercises. See how your body adapts. Get a little more dynamic and move around to engage more muscle groups.
THURSDAY: 4 miles easy.	If you feel you need a rest day mid week, you can skip today's miles. Don't fret about making the weekly mileage goal on a rest week; better to recoup!
FRIDAY: 6 miles easy pace. Core strength exercises.	Just keeping you moving with a few miles each day. Option: You could split this into two runs—3 miles in the morning and 3 miles later in the afternoon. This is a technique you can use as the mid-week miles increase.
SATURDAY: 10 miles easy pace.	This is your long run of the week and there are a few miles for tomorrow, but keep in mind this is your recovery week and rest is best! If you are not feeling recovered and ready to start another three-week building phase, then it is important to listen and scale this back. Better to have the motivation for next week!
SUNDAY: 5 miles steady.	Mix up the pace a bit from yesterday. Remember that this is the final day in your recovery week. Treat yourself well!

Week 5
Building (Speed) / Total Miles: 37–45, Long runs 12–14 and 8–10 miles

Jumping back into the miles! I hope you are rested up and ready to move daily. As we shift gears to a focus on speed, there is an introduction to the 5-minute repeat workout. This is one of my favorites. For the next three weeks, your weekly workout is going to focus on speed and leg turnover. The goal is setting a pace that is sustainable throughout the workout, while still pushing your edge. It may take a few attempts to figure out your ideal pace.

MONDAY: 6 miles easy.	This will warm you up for tomorrow's workout.
TUESDAY: 15 min warm up. 4 x 5 min repeats with 1-minute recovery. 15 min cool down. ~5-7 miles.	This is the workout I love and I hate. I dread going to the track (best place to manage pacing for me), because I know I need to work hard and it always keeps me honest. I love it because I always feel like I get a lot out of the effort when I am done. Give it a try. Be sure to read the description on page 49 (Run Workouts Descriptions) so that you figure out your pacing. Stay true to the 1-minute recovery. This workout will go by fast!
WEDNESDAY: 50 min cardio. Core strength exercises.	
THURSDAY: 6 miles. (2 warm up, 2 steady, 2 cool down.) ~6-8 miles.	This is a second workout for the week, but a pretty easy one. You can extend the middle steady miles to 3 or 4 if you are feeling good. Be sure to find a different pace for your warm up compared to the steady effort.
FRIDAY: Rest from running. Core strength exercises.	Keep in mind that you have two long runs coming up; do not do anything in your core workout that will make you too sore or stiff. Also, you are looking at a bit more of a time commitment this weekend for your long runs. Be sure to schedule appropriately so you get good rest Saturday night.
SATURDAY: 12–14-mile long run.	Back-to-back mileage over the weekends will get your body used to running on tired legs. As we move forward, these distances will be longer. It is great if you can mimic your racecourse terrain on your weekend trail runs.
SUNDAY: 8–10-mile long run.	

Week 6
Building (Speed) / Total Miles: 44–48, Long runs 12–14 and 8 miles

Remember, even though we are working on speed, it is important to mimic your goal racecourse during your weekend long runs. You want to keep your body working toward a familiarity with terrain that you will soon be racing over.

MONDAY: 5 miles easy. Core strength exercises.	Tomorrow will be a tough workout. Be sure this run gets you fired up and the core strength exercises leave something in your legs to be able to complete tomorrow's run strong!
TUESDAY: 15 min warm up. 5 x 5 min repeats with 1-minute recovery. 15 min cool down. ~6-8 miles.	Same workout as last week. Same day this week. Add another 5 minute repeat.
WEDNESDAY: Rest.	Last weekend's miles plus yesterday's workout is a solid accumulative effort and you might be feeling a little tired. Rest up today, stretch, hydrate, foam roll.
THURSDAY: 8 miles easy. (Run the middle 2–3 miles steady to mix up the pace.) Core strength exercises.	
FRIDAY: 5 miles steady.	
SATURDAY: 12–14-mile long run.	Have you experimented with hydration packs yet? (See Hydration & Nutrition Tips page 21 and Gear page 181) Your weekend long runs are the best time to figure out your gear. Plus, you should work on eating and drinking to help fuel your body and recover faster.
SUNDAY: 8-mile long run.	

Week 7

Building (Speed) / Total Miles: 38–50, Long runs 5–8 and 12–15 miles

Not only are you incorporating speed workouts, your mileage is now climbing out of your base range comfort zone. If your mileage has been steady shoot to hit the 50-mile mark this week. You have two speed workouts on your final week of this building phase. Tune into your body (keep writing down your thoughts) and how it responds to the workload. Are you tired? How is your appetite? Be sure to feed these cues—your body will tell you what it needs to continue training and to adapt to the increasing stress. Note: If you are more tired, get more sleep. Caffeine will not help your body adapt as much as a 15–20 minute nap, or an extra hour at night will.

MONDAY: Rest. Core strength exercises.	Today's workout is your opportunity to focus on a solid core strength routine. This week boosts two hard run workouts, so your second core strength day later in the week may be a bit lighter on the workload. Make today count.
TUESDAY: 5–6 miles easy.	To ready yourself for tomorrow's workout, throw a few 30-second surges into the later half of your workout. Three to four of them will feel good (recover at your easy pace in-between) and leave you ready for a hard effort tomorrow.
WEDNESDAY: 15 min warm up. 6 x 5 min repeats with 1-minute recovery. 15 min cool down. ~7-9 miles.	Six repeats, 30 minutes of hard running. It is key to find the pace that you can manage the entire workout! It might feel easy on the first two segments, but by the fourth you may be wishing you'd started a little more conservatively. Try to pace it out so you can finish your last lap at the same pace as your first.
THURSDAY: 5–6 miles easy OR 50 minutes cardio.	Take these miles super easy and use them to spin out your legs. OR if you prefer, opt for non-weight bearing movement to give you a bit more recovery. You have another speedy day tomorrow.
FRIDAY: 15 min warm up. PYRAMID Workout: 1, 2, 3, 2, 1 with equal recovery. 15 min cool down. ~4-6 miles.	You've done the pyramid workout before (week 3), but it was the only workout that week. This is following your tough Tuesday. The speed segments are shorter and should be a bit faster paced than Tuesday's repeats. Keep in mind you are looking forward to a recovery week next week. Use that as motivation to give a little more today.
SATURDAY: 5–8 miles easy. Core strength exercises.	Recover from your second speed workout, and know this is part of your back-to-back running over the weekend. This time the longer mileage is on day two.
SUNDAY: 12–15-mile long run.	Tally your miles for the week and tailor this run so that you hit the 50-mile week goal while staying in this suggested 12–15 mileage range. (I.e. do not run 20 miles today if you missed miles earlier this week.)

Week 8
Recovery / Total Miles: 27–33

With a little more time on your hands during this recovery week, read about gear options in Chapter 8. If you are already a pro at your current core strength routine, look into some new exercises that might up your game from the base you built. These lower mileage weeks also mean more time for social engagements. Make the most of this extra time by engaging with family and friends.

MONDAY: Rest.	Your motto for this week is "Rest is Best." Active recovery and daily runs will keep the consistency in your body and running awareness as a part of your life. If you are struggling to get out the door due to lack of motivation, this is the week to back off from "pushing through." There are workouts and long runs for which you will need the extra mojo in the future; this week is not the one to use up that important psyche.
TUESDAY: 4–6 miles easy. Core strength exercises.	It is okay to bump up the effort/weight/reps/sets on the core strength exercise workouts this week if you are feeling good about where you are recovery wise. With the extra time and less workload from running, your body can recover from the extra output. As always, use good form, work the whole body and put more emphasis on your legs one day.
WEDNESDAY: 5–7 miles easy.	Depending on how you are feeling, you can run the middle 2 miles at a steady pace for a change in turnover.
THURSDAY: 5 miles easy or 40–45 minutes cardio.	
FRIDAY: Rest from running. Core strength exercises.	
SATURDAY: 8-mile long run.	Today and tomorrow's runs are nothing crazy in terms of mileage. Just stay consistent and use these runs to recover. Think and feel "recovery" as you move through your miles.
SUNDAY: 5–7 mile easy run.	

Week 9
Building (Hills) / Total Miles: 38–45, Long runs 10-12 and 7-9 miles

We are now moving into hill workouts. These workouts will appear in the endurance phase, so you will see them again. As you plan your week, the responsibility falls on you to be honest with yourself. What kind of course are you training for? Look at the elevation profile and try to match your hill workouts to best prepare you for your race. Note: If you chose a relatively flat race course, hill workouts are still advantageous and helpful to your training. Be sure to find a runnable grade.

MONDAY: 4–6 miles easy. Core strength exercises.	
TUESDAY: 15 min warm up. PYRAMID HILL workout: 2, 4, 6, 4, 2 with equal recovery. 15 min cool down. ~6-8 miles.	This requires that you find a hill with a grade that you can run uninterrupted. After your warmup, find a pace that requires a steady effort while working to move uphill. If the grade (because of mimicking your race course) requires you to power hike (Tricks of the Trade, page 27), get in to it! Hands on knees, breathing hard and work to get up the hill efficiently! These are relatively short intervals with lots of recovery, so work at a challenging pace, one that you can sustain, but you feel like you are pushing to achieve. Recovery jog downhill in-between the efforts.
WEDNESDAY: 6 miles easy.	
THURSDAY: Rest or active recovery/ 35 min cardio.	
FRIDAY: 5–7 miles steady. Core strength exercises.	
SATURDAY: 10–12-mile long run.	Check in with your body and see how you have recovered from Tuesday's workout. If you feel ready, I challenge you to run these miles to match your racecourse profile. If you need to work on speed and turnover over rolling terrain, find a route that encourages it. If your climbs will be steep and require power hiking, take the time to find some mountains that force you to practice efficient form.
SUNDAY: 7–9 miles steady.	You do not have to work the hills as much today, but try to maintain a steady pace after yesterday's effort. No matter your racecourse, choose mellow, less technical terrain so that you can focus on maintaining a steady pace.

Week 10

Building (Hills) / Total Miles: 40-49, Long runs 12-14 and 10-12 miles

You are right in the middle of your hill phase. Keep strong and gain as much as you can from these workouts!

MONDAY: Rest.	Stretching and foam rolling will be helpful! You can move Tuesday's core strength exercises to today, if that works better for your schedule.
TUESDAY: 5 miles steady. Core strength exercises.	To ready yourself for tomorrow's workout, throw a few 30 second surges into the later half of your run; 3-4 will feel good (recover at your easy pace in-between) and leave you ready for a hard effort tomorrow.
WEDNESDAY: 15 min warm up. HILL Reverse Ladder 10, 8, 6, 3, 2, 1 with half time recovery. 15 min cool down. ~7-10 miles.	Normally you would climb the time ladder, but with this workout the longest repeat is first and they successively decrease in time (see Run Workout Descriptions, LADDER, page 48). Start with a pace that you can sustain and aim to finish the last few with more intensity. Note that the recovery time is half of the interval time. Recovery jog downhill in-between the efforts.
THURSDAY: Rest/active recovery 40 min cardio.	An extra rest day this week, which means you run more mileage on the days you do run.
FRIDAY: 6-8 miles easy. Core strength exercises.	
SATURDAY: 12-14-mile long run.	Long run of the week.
SUNDAY: 10-12-mile long run.	Back up yesterday's long run with another to top off your weekly mileage.

Week 11

Building (Hills) / Total Miles: 48–57, Long runs 18–20 and 14–16 miles

You are looking at a pretty solid mileage week, with a tough speed workout on hump day. Learn to love this workout. It is a super beneficial one for pacing and training your threshold. It is hard and it hurts sometimes, but in the 60–90 minutes that it takes you to do it, you will feel like you got more out of the time than a 3–4 hour run. And recovery comes next week, so you totally have this.

MONDAY: 45 min cardio. Core strength exercises.	If it makes sense to switch Monday's and Tuesday's workouts, that is an option.
TUESDAY: 5–8 miles easy.	Getting your legs back under you for tomorrow's speed workout.
WEDNESDAY: 15–20 min warm up. 5 x 5 min HILL with 1 min recovery. 15 min cool down. ~6-8 miles.	You have done this as a speed workout. Now take it to a hill. Having a consistent runnable hill might be the best for this one (even if your course requires you to power hike). Working on your running stamina on hills is always a great way to build confidence and strength. This will be tough with only one-minute recovery. Plan a little post-run reward for getting through this one!
THURSDAY: 5 miles easy. Core strength exercises.	Definitely move today. These miles might feel a little funny, and your legs may be heavy. Be sure to keep the miles easy and shake out yesterday's workout. Take note of how your body is feeling for the core strength exercise workout. If you are okay, work on legs a bit more than normal. You have a rest day tomorrow.
FRIDAY: Rest.	Prepare for some LONG miles this weekend!!!
SATURDAY: 18–20 miles.	This is a jump in your long run mileage followed by another big day tomorrow. Take note. Listen to your body. Choose terrain that you are ready for. Prepare for more time out on the trails and plan for the necessary recovery nutrition so that you are ready for more on Sunday!
SUNDAY: 14–16-mile long run.	You can do it—the legs might be a little tired and/or stiff from this week and yesterday's effort. Take your time to warm up, fuel, hydrate and move through these fun miles. After this it is all about recovery!

Week 12
Recovery / Total Miles: 19–28

You are coming off a couple of solid blocks: speed and hills. You have also just finished some of your longest training runs of the plan. Congrats! We are midway to your goal! I encourage you to look ahead and see that the remainder of the plan continues to build. You have a solid base of miles and your body is tuned to receive the coming weeks of training. With that in mind, take a breather this week. Get life in order to be able to accommodate the longer training hours that will be a significant part of the next three months. Build up that mojo and get excited! There is a lot of exploring, both on the trails and within you, to come.

MONDAY: Rest.	You've definitely earned this one! Hopefully you feel ready to chill this week. Take note of how you are feeling each day. Are you tired early in the week? Does that improve by Wednesday or Thursday? How about your appetite? You may be super hungry even by mid-week. Your body is likely making up for the potential caloric deficit accumulated last week. As we get into longer training miles your need for sleep and calories will continue to increase. It is good to pay attention to these needs now so that you continue to be aware later.
TUESDAY: 3-5 miles easy. Core strength exercises.	
WEDNESDAY: 5 miles easy or 45-60 min cardio.	Stretch and foam roll too!
THURSDAY: Rest from running. Core strength exercises.	Hopefully your body is starting to feel recovered and you can put in a good effort on the core strength exercises workout today.
FRIDAY: 5-8 miles as you feel.	
SATURDAY: 6-10 miles easy.	
SUNDAY: Rest.	

Week 13
Building (Endurance) / Total Miles: 51–62, Long runs 8–10 and 18 miles

The endurance phase will be tough. It should be! You've signed up to run a 50-mile or 100K race! You want to be ready. Staying consistent plays a major roll in the coming weeks, as the daily running will build your body to handle the longer miles. Often times you will see both speed and hill workouts scheduled. Having multiple workouts in a week means that you need to spend just as much time managing your body and tending to aches and small pains before they cause problems. Foam rolling, stretching (see Recovery Movement, EXTRA PIECES, page 230) and of course your core strength exercises are huge factors in keeping your body healthy as you build these miles.

*Note: If you plan to run a 50K as part of your training, be sure to use Alterntive week 15 this build phase.

MONDAY: 5 miles steady. Core strength exercises.	Now you have played around with core strength exercise workouts and know how to get a full body workout. Make sure to keep doing the exercises you don't really like (those are the ones you may need the most!) and piece together workouts that increase overall strength.
TUESDAY: 15–20 min warm up. PYRAMID SPEED workout: 1, 2, 3, 4, 3, 2, 1 with equal recovery. 15 min cool down. ~7-10 miles.	This is your speed workout of the week. Less technical terrain is best so you can work on turnover. Make these intervals a little quicker than normal, especially the 1- and 2-minute ones. Run smart and use good form!
WEDNESDAY: Rest from running. Core strength exercises.	Pay attention to your legs after the speed session yesterday. For the core strength exercise workout, shoot for 45 minutes–1 hour and hit the whole body. Just be careful not to tweak or aggravate anything that might be tender from your pace yesterday.
THURSDAY: 5–8 miles easy.	Keep in mind you have a tough workout tomorrow!
FRIDAY: 15–20 min warm up. HILL workout: 1) 3 x 6–8 minutes uphill power hiking w/ 3 min recovery between. 2) 10 min easy run. 3) 5 x 30 second uphill surge w/1 min–90 seconds recovery. 15 min cool down. ~8-11 miles.	Hopefully you have your legs back under you and are ready for this one. There are three pieces to this workout (besides the WU & CD.) 1) Find a steep grade that requires you to power hike at a sustainable pace. 2) After the repeats, run easy for about 10 minutes. 3) Find a runnable grade that gets your attention, you want to be all out on the 30-second repeats and fully recover in between (you can take more recovery time than assigned if you need). Hopefully you can run without interruptions. Make it happen!
SATURDAY: 8–10 miles easy.	This should feel good after yesterday's hard effort.
SUNDAY: 18-mile long run.	Okay. You might be tired. It's been a tough week. You've got a day off from running tomorrow (don't forget core strength exercises though!). Do not do anything that is going to injure you today (ever). When you start a run tired, it is good to use these miles for mental training. Focus on hydration and nutrition as aides to get you through. Taking in a few more calories than you are used to might make this a little easier. Definitely recover well afterward.

Week 14
Building (Endurance) / Total Miles: 55–65, Long runs 18–20 and 10–12 miles

The 5-minute repeats workout is back this week! Love to hate it, hate to love it. It's awesome and will do wonders as you recover from it. Your Saturday long run should be hilly, so think ahead about location and possible travel time if necessary.

MONDAY: No run. Core strength exercises.	Core strength exercises are your only workout today. I hope it is a good one for you! If you feel like you need a complete REST day, then take today off and move the core strength exercise workout to tomorrow in addition to the miles. Sometimes a full rest day can do wonders.
TUESDAY: 6–8 miles easy.	
WEDNESDAY: 15 min warm up. 5–6 x 5 min with 1 min recovery. 15–20 min cool down. ~8–10 miles.	You have done this one before and you will do it again. Find that steady, strong pace that gets you through all of the repeats. Be sure to recover well after this! Hydrate, eat, sleep!
THURSDAY: 8–10 miles steady.	This is a mid-week long run and might be a little tough after yesterday's workout. You can switch with Friday's schedule, just be aware of your weekend mileage.
FRIDAY: 5 miles easy. Core strength exercises.	
SATURDAY: 18–20-mile long run.	You do not have a hill workout this week, so make your weekend runs hilly and similar to your racecourse profile if possible. You should work the hills a bit, try to think about how you want to feel and perform in your race while running or power-hiking uphill as well as your speed for down hills.
SUNDAY: 10–12-mile run.	Do not slack on these miles. This is your back-to-back. You want these miles to feel like miles 35–42 of your 50-mile race.

Week 15
Building (Endurance) / Total Miles: 57–68, Long runs 20–22 and 9–11 miles

You have been running strong for a while and this is the last week of this first endurance building phase. If you are waning a bit read Train Your Brain, Q & A #2, page 37. You can look forward to a recovery week next week! We are getting into your biggest weekly mileage, which means a lot of things: more time on your feet, more energy output, bigger appetite and extra sleep to recover properly. Budget your time wisely and prepare meals and gear bags ahead of time to save you time and ensure good recovery fuel and hydration.

MONDAY: Rest.	Finally a full rest day!
TUESDAY: 9-mile run. Warm up for the first 2–3 miles. Keep the middle 3 miles steady. Cool down the last 3 miles.	This is a big run for your first run of the week. It falls this way so that you can get in two good efforts during the week in addition to the longer mileage runs this weekend. Really warm up and cool down at a comfortable pace. Push the middle 3–4 so that you feel your effort (aka tempo). These middle miles are your speed miles this week.
WEDNESDAY: 5–7 miles steady. Core strength exercises.	You have core strength exercises on either side of your hill workout this week, so think about which day makes the most sense to put the emphasis on your legs, or if you want to just go for full body both days.
THURSDAY: 15–20 min warm up. HILL Workout: 1) 4 x 6 min with 3 min recovery. 2) 5 minutes easy. 3) 3 x 2 min with 1 min recovery. 5 minutes easy. 3 x 30 seconds with full recovery (90 seconds). 15 min cool down. ~9-12 miles.	Adding another segment to this familiar workout (like Week 13's 3-part hill workout). Continue to increase your pace as you move through. For the second set—3 x 2 min—try to pick up the pace compared to how you were doing the 6-minute intervals. And for the final 30-second repeats give your all.
FRIDAY: 5–7 miles easy. Core strength exercises.	
SATURDAY: 20–22-mile long run.	The workouts from this week are in your legs. You have done tougher workouts than you did this week but it is this weekend that will add up and you will feel it. These two long back-to-backs are the bulk of the week. Try to keep the middle 5–8 miles of today at a good up-tempo pace. Opting for a course with a good elevation profile (mimics your racecourse) is also always something to consider.
SUNDAY: 9–11-mile run.	You have a full rest day tomorrow and you are going into a recovery week! Make these miles count.

Week 15 Alternate
50k race + 38–45 miles = 69–76 miles, Long runs 31 and 10–12 miles

If you have opted to incorporate a 50 km race into your 50-mile training schedule, follow this week's workouts and have a blast racing over the weekend. Keep in mind that you are training through this race which means you are not tapering as much and your legs will have more miles in them going into the race than usual. You might not feel your spunkiest or speediest, but remember it is training. Read through Chapter Eleven, Race Day Preparations: Ready? Set?, page 199, and utilize the Race Packing List, EXTRA PIECES, page 226.

MONDAY: 5 miles easy. Core strength exercises.	Make today's core strength exercise workout quality. That does not mean you have to lift heavy weights or do repeats until failure, just give your exercises the time they need to feel like you worked all of your muscle groups and got a good workout.
TUESDAY: 15–20 min warm up. SPEED workout—either PYRAMID SPEED workout: 1, 2, 3, 4, 3, 2, 1 with equal recovery. OR 4 x 5 min with 1 min recovery. 15 min cool down. ~6-8 miles.	I want you to choose a speed workout that sounds good to you. I've suggested either the pyramid speed workout or the 5-minute intervals. Aim for 20 minutes of higher intensity running spread out over the intervals. Keep your weekend race in mind—use that as focus to run smart and feel how you want to feel while racing on Saturday. Likewise, recover well after!
WEDNESDAY: 12–15-mile mid-week long run.	You can split this into two runs. 6-8 in the morning and the remainder in the evening.
THURSDAY: Rest from running. Core strength exercises.	Do not do anything too crazy with your legs to make you sore or tired for the weekend.
FRIDAY: 5 miles easy with 4 x 100 m strides at end.	Easy miles to work out any bugs before your race. Use the strides to visualize how you want to feel when you are finishing tomorrow.
SATURDAY: 50 km training race.	Utilize this race to prep for your 50-miler. This is a great opportunity to practice/refresh how you want to move through aid stations, interact with your crew and pace yourself in a race situation. If you are curious about a different race strategy (like going out hard when you typically take it easy, or visa versa, or surging at mile 20 for a strong finish) this would be a good place to test it if you feel your training has you prepared for that kind of effort. You have miles to run tomorrow; do not go too crazy. Good luck!
SUNDAY: 10–12-mile long run easy pace.	This is a little longer than a normal shakeout run and if you raced too hard yesterday, this might feel impossible. Give your body a chance, take the time to warm up and see if you can work the kinks out and start to feel better.

Week 16

Recovery / Total Miles: 19–24

This recovery week should be well-timed. REST UP! Let all of that work absorb into your body. Continue to fuel and hydrate appropriately so your body can heal from the training and get stronger. You have one more endurance phase that you want to be ready for. This downtime is the preparation you need to be able to charge again.

MONDAY: Rest.	Two full rest days this week; one to start the week and one to finish it off. If it feels like you need an additional rest day, either Wednesday or Thursday would be a good one to swap out. You could always move the Wednesday or Thursday workout to Sunday.
TUESDAY: 3–5 miles easy. Core strength exercises.	
WEDNESDAY: 5 miles easy or 45–60 min cardio.	Do one of these today and the other tomorrow.
THURSDAY: 5 miles easy or 45–60 min cardio.	Do the opposite of what you did yesterday.
FRIDAY: 6–8 miles as you feel. Core strength exercises.	Hopefully you are feeling more recovered and strong. If so, this would be a good day to have a solid training session for core strength exercises.
SATURDAY: 5–6 miles easy.	
SUNDAY: Rest.	If you can, do not think about running AT ALL today. I think it is good to take a mental break. Do not train physically or mentally today, just be.

Week 17
Building (Endurance) / Total Miles: 61–69, Long runs 25 and 14 miles

You will see your highest mileage weeks in this next phase. The weekends will be occupied with running and recovering. In other words, it is time to focus. As your weekend back-to-back runs get longer and longer it is a good time to really start tuning in to the mental aspect of your training. Running ultras is very physical, and it is pretty straightforward on how to train that piece. It is the mental aspect that will see you through to the ultra finish line. Try some of the mental training tips in Train Your Brain, page 33 during your long runs this weekend and in the coming weeks.

MONDAY: 4–6 miles easy. Core strength exercises.	The miles are to warm you up for the speed workout tomorrow.
TUESDAY: 15 min warm up. 6 x 5 min with 1 min recovery. 15 min cool down. ~7–10 miles.	You will see this workout every week for this phase, adding one interval each week. Stick to your pace through the intervals. Try to be super consistent and finish as strong as you start! If you raced week 15, you may need additional recovery before jumping into a workout. You can swap this with Thursday's miles and move Thursday's core workout to Wednesday.
WEDNESDAY: 6-mile steady run.	Flush out yesterday's workout.
THURSDAY: 5–8 miles easy. Core strength exercises.	Get ready for some BIG miles this weekend.
FRIDAY: Rest.	There is not a hill workout this week, but I highly recommend planning the weekend to mimic your racecourse. If there are hills on race day, make one or both of your weekend runs match the race profile the best you can.
SATURDAY: 25-mile long run.	Today and tomorrow are two significant back-to-back runs. Plan on these taking a significant amount of your time, not only to run, but also to prepare gear, food and recovery eats for, commute, and recover. Do not be surprised if all you want to do come Sunday afternoon (assuming you run in the morning) is take a nap. If you can, I highly encourage it. 20–30 minutes will do wonders for your recovery and help you finish the day with a smile.
SUNDAY: 14-mile long run.	

Week 18
Building (Endurance) / Total Miles: 64–75, Long runs 25–28 and 12–15 miles

Moving in to week two of a three week building phase can be mentally tough. You are in the thick of the mileage, that is, you already have a week's worth built up, and have more to go. This is where the mental training comes in. Remember the mental training techniques (Chapter Five, Train Your Brain, page 33) to work through these miles. You will train your mind for the tough times or low points that could show up during your race. Be kind to yourself, but also test your edge and learn what you are made of.

MONDAY: 5 miles easy. Core strength exercises.	
TUESDAY: 15 min warm up. 7 x 5 min with 1 min recovery. 15 min cool down. ~8-10 miles.	
WEDNESDAY: 8-11 miles steady.	Another mid-week long run. Remember you can split the miles into two runs. Also, if you are fatigued from yesterday's workout, you can switch the rest day to today and run longer tomorrow. Just keep in mind that switch will put your long miles closer to your big weekend.
THURSDAY: Rest.	
FRIDAY: 6 miles easy. Core strength exercises.	Gauge how you are feeling after Wednesday's run and know that you are running long tomorrow. Think about giving yourself as much recovery time as possible. Hint: Do both of these workouts in the morning so you have the remainder of the day to hydrate, fuel, rest and prep for tomorrow.
SATURDAY: 25-28-mile long run.	Use the mileage ranges on these two runs to achieve your weekly goal. You do not want to total much more than 75 miles this week because you have to build again next week. RACE PLANNING: Use these weekend's long runs to prep yourself for the race. Running on similar terrain is awesome! Also think about testing all of your gear before the race. All clothing. All nutrition. Have everything dialed!! (See Race Day Preparations, Chapter Eleven, page 199.)
SUNDAY: 12-15-mile long run.	

Week 19
Building (Endurance) / Total Miles: 75–80, Long runs 28–30 and 15 miles

You should be focused on eating, sleeping and running. There will be some down time, of course, but it might be your best plan to focus on your training runs and not overbook yourself otherwise.

MONDAY: Rest.	
TUESDAY: 5 miles easy. Core strength exercises.	Pay attention to your recovery from last weekend. Will you be ready for tomorrow's workout? Do what is necessary to ensure that you are.
WEDNESDAY: 15 min warm up. 7–8 x 5 min with 1 min recovery. 15 min cool down. ~10–13 miles.	The last two repeats of this workout are always tough for me. I know people that do upwards of 10–12 repeats, but 8 repeats seem to be a worthy workout for me. If you do the math, this is 40 minutes at a much faster than race pace effort. (10 would be 50 minutes and 12 an hour.) As race distances get longer and times get more competitive, the training bar rises. The most important thing you can do is maintain your pace for all of the repeats and feel good after the workout. You have your longest block of mileage this week, so you definitely want to do this workout no later than Wednesday, so that you have the next two days to recover.
THURSDAY: 5 miles steady.	You can add some core strength exercises if you are feeling it. Look ahead, the next three days are back-to-back-to-back! Plan ahead...
FRIDAY: 12 miles steady.	Pack your kit for tomorrow's run. Plan out a few food options that you think you would like to eat during the race and try them out while running. Consider the clothing you want to wear in your race and run in these pieces. It is best to dial in as much as possible prior to your race so that the only "new" experience is going your farthest distance to date.
SATURDAY: 28–30-mile long run.	This is your longest mileage on a back-to-back weekend. Be sure to take really good care. This is the weekend to focus on running, eating and sleeping. Minimize extra work and social activities.
SUNDAY: 15-mile long run.	

Week 20
Recovery / Total Miles: 28–35

We are getting close now. Can you believe that this is your last recovery week (besides your taper) before your race? It is exciting to think about! Don't get too amped just yet. There are still a couple of weeks to fine tune your dialed machine and then your taper period will feel a lot like a long recovery week. The cool thing about your taper is that by now you have taught your body how to recover and absorb the training. You know how to recharge and your muscles bounce back faster so that you can perform better and stronger for the next phase, or in this case, the race. Keep this in mind as you recover this week, pay attention to how your body turns around from tired to recovered.

MONDAY: Rest.	The layout of this recovery week should feel pretty familiar by now. I hope the familiarity works for you. If there are some runs or workouts that you prefer during your recovery week, I definitely encourage you to do what feels good. Keep in mind that "Rest is Best" this week.
TUESDAY: 3–5 miles easy. Core strength exercises.	It is possible, and likely, that you will still feel the effects of your long weekend of running. Ease into these miles, or take another rest day. Recovery is key this week!
WEDNESDAY: 6–8 miles easy or 60–75 min cardio.	While you have a little extra time this week, review the previous four months of your training plan and set in your mind the significance of the training you have done up to this point. Relive a few of your more challenging workouts or long runs and reflect on the lessons you learned about yourself. These are the pieces that will give you confidence in your race.
THURSDAY: Rest.	You can switch today's rest day for Sunday's miles if you would like to have a full day off over the weekend.
FRIDAY: 6 miles as you feel. Core strength exercises.	
SATURDAY: 8–10 miles easy.	
SUNDAY: 5–6 miles easy.	If you ran these miles on Thursday, then be sure to rest up today.

Week 21
Fine-Tuning / Total Miles: 62–66. Last back-to-back 25 and 12 miles

Fine tuning is as it sounds. Fine-tune you. Dial in your gear. (Read Race Preparations: Ready? Set? Chapter Eleven). You have learned a lot about your body up to this point; now apply it in these next two weeks. Do the workouts that give you the best feeling and results. Eat the foods and time your recovery so that you feel dialed before, during and after every run. Read through the course description, visualize and project your best race. Make your body work for you. Make your mind work for you.

MONDAY: Rest from running. Core strength exercises.	
TUESDAY: 7-9 miles easy.	Throw in a couple of pickups of various time durations (2-6 minutes) throughout the run. Quicken your pace in preparation for tomorrow. Keep a good pace and cool down the final 1-2 miles.
WEDNESDAY: 15 min warm up. SPEED 5-7 x 5 min with 1 min recovery. 15 min cool down. OR 15 min warm up. HILL workout: 1, 3, 5, 7, 5, 3, 1 with half time recovery. 15 min cool down. ~8-11 miles.	You have an option today: speed or hills. Pick one. Do not do both. If you pick speed today, be sure to make Friday's run hilly and run/power hike with intention. If you pick hills today, run a speedier course Friday and throw in a good tempo (15-20 minutes) and a couple of surges (3-6 x 1-2 minutes). *Note–look ahead at Tuesday, week 22. My comments there might influence today's choice.
THURSDAY: 3 easy miles. Core strength exercises.	
FRIDAY: 7 miles steady.	Be sure to read the notes from Wednesday. Make this a good workout type run, opposite of what you chose Wednesday.
SATURDAY: 25-mile long run.	Dial it in! This weekend is your last to test any new gear you are considering for race day. If you want to completely geek out, you could even practice an aid station run through with your crew. All of the preparation will help you plan what to pack. Start making a list (or use the Race Packing list, EXTRA PIECES on page 226), and note the items in your running pack that you might not think of later. It is best to write down everything while you are using it (or just after) rather than trying to think of what you need two days later.
SUNDAY: 12-mile long run.	

Week 22

Fine-Tuning / Total Miles: 43–51. Last long run 18–22 miles.

This week is about dialing back the mileage, putting in quality efforts when you run and maintaining the rest of the week. It is time to start feeling confident, strong and ready. You do not have to be completely there yet, but you should feel your body working toward that final preparation.

MONDAY: 5 miles easy. Core strength exercises.	If 50 minutes of cardio sounds more appealing on either Monday or Wednesday, then that can be helpful active non-weight bearing movement.
TUESDAY: 15 min warm up. 6–8 x 5 min with 1 min recovery. 15 min cool down. OR 15 min warm up. HILL workout: 1, 3, 5, 7, 5, 3, 1 with half time recovery. 15 min cool down. ~9-11 miles.	If you opted for hills in week 21, shoot for speed, 7–8 x 5-minute repeats this week. If you chose speed last week, then do the hill workout. *IF* you really love the 5-minute repeat workout and feel the benefits **and** you think it will serve you best for your race preparations, then go for your best. Do one more repeat than you did last week and work hard to maintain an even pace over the entire workout. Regardless, what you choose today is your last hard workout.
WEDNESDAY: 4–6 miles easy. Core strength exercises.	If you are really into the core strength exercise workouts (I hope you are!) and enjoy putting time into getting stronger (sweet!), please make this your last hard core strength exercises workout. You have core strength exercises in the taper weeks, but that should be body weight exercises only, and nothing that will make you sore.
THURSDAY: Rest.	
FRIDAY: 7 miles hilly and steady.	
SATURDAY: 18–22-mile long run.	This is your last long run! Make this a GREAT one! Test all of your race gear and your nutrition plan. Feel awesome afterwards … recover smart.
SUNDAY: Rest.	If you can, do not think about running AT ALL today. Do not train physically or mentally today, just be.

Week 23
Taper / Total Miles: 24–32

This might feel like a long taper, but I think it will be worth it. You have put in some amazing miles leading up to this point and now it is time for your body to do what it has learned throughout this program—that is to recover.

MONDAY: Rest/active recovery.	If you haven't already, now would be a great time to start dialing in your crew or drop bags. Whatever resupply system you are going to use for the race, figure it out now. It is best to work on these things sooner than later. Having this taken care of will ease your mind. I have offered up thoughts for crew preparations on page 173 and drop bag packing on page 178.
TUESDAY: 3–5 miles steady. Core strength exercises.	If 40 minutes of cardio sounds more appealing on either Tuesday or Thursday (or both!), then that can be helpful active non-weight bearing movement. Remember to keep your core strength exercises workouts effective, but do not over do it.
WEDNESDAY: 15 min warm up. 4–5 x 5 min with 1 min recovery. 15 min cool down. ~5–7 miles.	This should feel easy and you should start to feel like you are going to be ready for the race weekend. This is a good time to check in on what you need to be rested and primed for race weekend.
THURSDAY: 3–5 miles easy. Core strength exercises.	If 40 minutes of cardio sounds more appealing, then that can be helpful active non-weight bearing movement. Remember to keep your core strength exercises workouts effective, but do not over do it.
FRIDAY: Rest.	
SATURDAY: 8–10-mile trail run.	Run within yourself. Have fun! Visualize what you are going to feel like next week at this time. You might try starting at the same time as the race starts (only if you can ensure a good night's sleep on either side). It would be a good way to ready your system.
SUNDAY: 5 miles.	Take this easy. Spin out your legs. This is just to keep you from starting the taper tantrums (Train Your Brain, Chapter Five, Question #4, page 38) too early. If you feel like rest would be better, then go for it! A little active recovery or cardio could also be a good option.

Week 24

50M RACE WEEK! Taper and rest up! 60–63 miles including race

Are the taper tantrums setting in for you? Keep calm and train your mind. The mental aspect is what is going to get you through. These final days before the race, when you are feeling antsy and would prefer to just run, focus your mind and visualize a great run this weekend. The excess energy will be much better spent training your mind than wasting it on excess movement. Remember there is no training run you can do this week that will make your race better, only rest, sleep and good nutrition/hydration will give you the positive impacts you seek.

MONDAY: Rest.	You can do some of your favorite core strength exercises, but do not do anything to make you sore or that you cannot recover from.
TUESDAY: 10 min warm up. 3–5 x 2 min with 1 min jog/recovery. 10 min cool down. ~4-5 miles.	This is just to make you feel good and fast. Remember, nothing you do this week will have time to settle in your body and make you have a better race. The sole purpose is movement to keep you calm.
WEDNESDAY: 3-5 miles easy.	This can be a rest day or 30–40 minute cardio workout. Really listen to what will be best for you!
THURSDAY: Rest.	Train your mind. Re-read the visualization segment in Train Your Brain Chapter 5, page 33.
FRIDAY: 3 miles easy. 4 x 100m strides.	This is so that you sweat and work out some of the kinks before your race. Remember I feel it is best to move the day before you put out your best effort. You might feel slow and a little clunky after so much rest. Remember all of your visualization and be positive. Believe that this is working out the tiny hitches and tomorrow will feel amazing.
SATURDAY: 50-Mile Race	Very exciting! Race day is here! Please read page 205 for my last little tidbits ... I am excited for you and, more importantly, I hope you are excited for you.
SUNDAY: CELEBRATE!	

FIRST 100M

Description: Consistent runner.

Mileage average: 50 miles/week for the last 3 months

Race history: Ran a couple 50ks and/or 50 milers in the last 2 years

Minimum training time per week available: 12 hours/week

Training period: 8-12 months*

Every life experience will help you succeed in your 100-mile race.

Training Plan Notes:

This plan jumps right in assuming your mileage base is consistent and your body is healthy and recovered from any long efforts. This is a 48-week plan. You do not want to burnout midway through because you did not recover sufficiently before starting.

You are committing a year to training for what might be the biggest physical challenge of your life. To focus your training and help differentiate some of the phases, I include speed, hill and endurance phases as shown in the 50k and 50-mile plans. Here, you have more time and the ability to customize your schedule based on your race goals. There are options to move building blocks, depending on what you think you need. In training and racing shorter ultra distances, you have learned what works for you. Now I challenge you to apply those lessons to training for 100 miles. One difference is that rest and recovery between your last hard training effort and race day is even more crucial. The more recovery you can put in the bank the entire month prior to your 100, the better the last 20 miles will feel.

→ Weeks 1–7 of the 100-mile plan closely mimic weeks 9–15 of the 50-mile plan.

→ Month 4 is less cumulative mileage than the previous month, but you have the intensity of the race miles.

→ In week 41, if you feel you need one more week to feel more recovered after your race, I suggest following the plan written for week 46 instead and use the extra time to get back into running (about 45–50 miles). To finish out the calendar bump ahead what I wrote for week 41 to week 42, 42 to 43, 43 to 44, 44 to 45, 45 to 46, then jump back in to 47 as it is. Either plan will work; it is up to you to figure out which is best for you. (You can see this written out on the Distances Summary page and the optional W41–48 schedule). Note that this alternate moves 10 miles from month 12 to month 11. This might be something to consider—a few less miles closer to your 100-mile race might be just the ticket for your preparedness.

→ If 12 months isn't feasible for your first 100-mile race I suggest a minimum 8 months of focused training. This will give you time to learn about your body and your gear, and to train your endurance and recovery systems properly.

→ If you recently (within the last two months) ran a 50k or 50-mile race you can start at Month 4.

→ If your monthly mileage average is around 180–200 miles (for two–three months) you could start at Month 4.

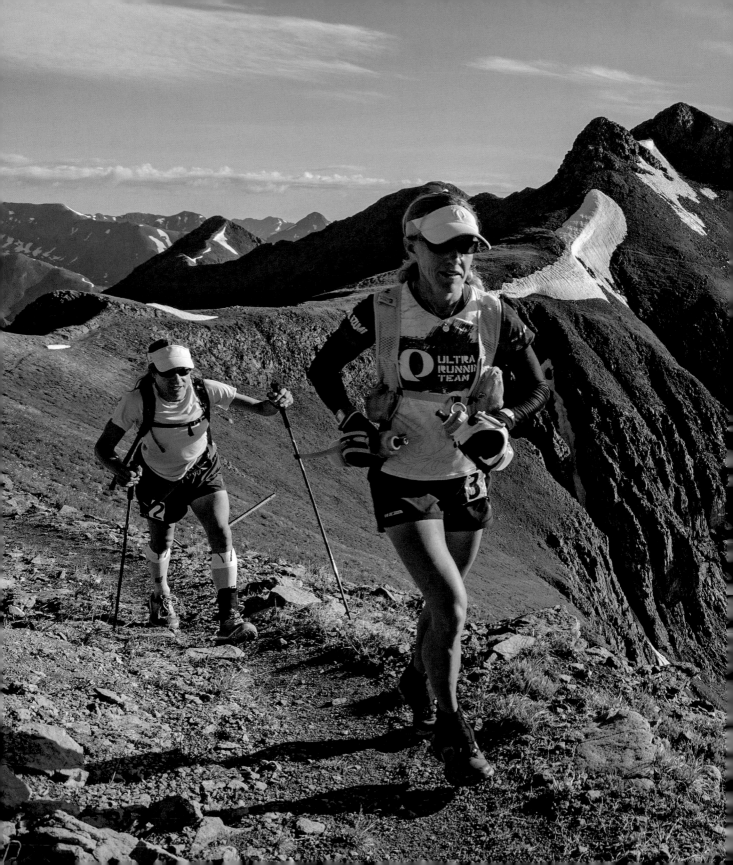

100-MILE TRAINING PLAN

Monthly/Weekly Overview

If you prefer to train by time instead of miles, figure out your average minute/mile pace and multiply it by the scheduled miles. Ex1: 5 miles easy. Your easy pace is 10 minutes/mile. 5 x 10 = 50 minutes of easy running. Ex2: 8 miles steady. Your steady pace is 8:30. 8 x 8.5 = 68 minutes of steady running.

MONTH 1: TOTAL 149–186 MILES

Week 1 - Building 39–50 miles, long runs 10–12 and 7–9 miles

Week 2 - Building 41–50 miles, long runs 12–14 and 10–12 miles

Week 3 - Building 50–58 miles, long runs 18 and 14 miles

Week 4 - Recovery 19–28 miles

MONTH 2: TOTAL 181–212 MILES

Week 5 - Building (Hills) 51–59 miles, long runs 10 and 18 miles

Week 6 - Building (Hills) 50–61 miles, long runs 18–20 and 6–8 miles

Week 7 - Building (Hills) 56–63 miles, long runs 20–22 and 9–11 miles

Week 8 - Recovery 24–29 miles

MONTH 3: TOTAL 219–251 MILES

Week 9 - Building (Speed) 56–66 miles, long runs 18 and 10–14 miles

Week 10 - Building (Speed) 68–72 miles, long runs 20 and 15 miles

Week 11 - Building (Speed) 63–78 miles, long runs 22–24 and 15–18 miles

Week 12 - Recovery 32–35 miles

MONTH 4 (50K OR 50M RACE): TOTAL 197–241 MILES

Week 13 - Building (Speed) 59–68 miles, long runs 18–22 and 10–12 miles

Week 14 - 48–61 miles. Run 30–35 miles early in week, start 50 km taper by Thursday. OR run 25–30 miles early in week, start 50M taper by Wednesday.

Week 15 - 58 or 77 miles. Taper 27 miles during week + 50 km or 50 M race (part of training)

Week 16 - Recovery 32–35 miles

MONTH 4 ALTERNATE (NO RACE): TOTAL 226–261 MILES

Week 13 - Building (Speed) 59–68 miles, long runs 18–22 and 10–12 miles

Week 14 - Building (Speed) 64–76 miles, long runs 25 and 10–13 miles

Week 15 - Building (Speed) 71–82 miles, long runs 26–30 and 10–12 miles

Week 16 - Recovery 32–35 miles

MONTH 5: TOTAL 232–267 MILES

Week 17 - Building (Endurance) 54–67 miles, long runs 18–22 and 10–12 miles

Week 18 - Building (Endurance) 67–79 miles, long runs 13–15 and 22–24 miles

Week 19 - Building (Endurance) 79–86 miles, long runs 28–30 and 10–12 miles

Week 20 - Recovery 32–35 miles

MONTH 6: TOTAL 260–285 MILES

Week 21 - Building (Endurance) 71–72 miles, long runs 26–28 and 10–12 miles

Week 22 - Building (Endurance) 76–86 miles, long runs 28 and 15–18 miles

Week 23 - Building (Endurance) 80–90 miles, long runs 28–30 and 18 miles

Week 24 - Recovery 33–37 miles

MONTH 7: TOTAL 271–298 MILES

Week 25 - Building (Hills) 72–80 miles, long runs 30–34 and 10 miles

Week 26 - Building (Hills) 80–88 miles, long runs 40 and 8–10 miles

Week 27 - Building (Hills) 84–90 miles, long runs 45 and 8–10 miles

Week 28 - Recovery 35–40 miles

MONTH 8 (RACE): TOTAL 232–282 MILES

Week 29 - Building (Endurance) 63–82 miles, long runs 25–28 and 12–14 miles

Week 30 - Race Prep 50–58 miles

Week 31 - Race Prep 37–43 miles + Run 50M to 100K Race

Week 32 - Recovery 32–37 miles

MONTH 8 ALTERNATE (NO RACE): TOTAL 269–313 MILES

Week 29 - Building (Endurance) 63–82 miles, long runs 25–28 and 12–14 miles

Week 30 - Building (Endurance) 83–94 miles, long runs 35–40 and 8–12 miles

Week 31 - Building (Endurance) 91–100 miles, long runs 42–45 and 10–12 miles

Week 32 - Recovery 32–37 miles

MONTH 9: TOTAL 183–215 MILES

Week 33 - Recovery total 50–54 miles, long runs 10–12 and 8 miles

Week 34 - Recovery 49–58 miles, long runs 15–18 and 10 miles

Week 35 - Recovery 52–66 miles, long runs 18–22 and 10–14 miles

Week 36 - Recovery 32–37 miles

MONTH 10: TOTAL 288–319 MILES

Week 37 - Building (Endurance) 86–94 miles, long runs 30–34 and 12–14 miles

Week 38 - Building (Endurance) 85–96 miles, long runs 35 and 20–25 miles

Week 39 - Building (Endurance) 82–94 miles, long runs 35–40 and 8–10 miles

Week 40 - Recovery 35 miles

MONTH 11: TOTAL 209–243 MILES

Week 41 - Building (Speed) 50–58 miles, long runs 15–18 and 8 miles

Week 42 - Building (Speed) 61–70 miles, long runs 18–22 and 10–12 miles

Week 43 - Building (Speed) 63–75 miles, long runs 25–28 and 12 miles

Week 44 - Recovery 35–40 miles

MONTH 12: TOTAL 209–225 MILES

Week 45 - Prepping 50–54 miles, long runs 16 and 18 miles

Week 46 - Prepping 40–46 miles, long runs 12–14 and 8 miles

Week 47 - Tapering 24–32 miles

Week 48 - **Race 100 Miles!**

ALTERNATE FINAL 8 WEEKS

MONTH 11: TOTAL 214–249 MILES

Week 41 - Prepping 40–46 miles, long runs 12–14 and 8 miles

Week 42 - Building (Speed) 50–58 miles, long runs 15–18 and 10–12 miles

Week 43 - Building (Speed) 61–70 miles, long runs 25–28 and 12 miles

Week 44 - Building (Speed) 63–75 miles

MONTH 12: TOTAL 209–226 MILES

Week 45 - Recovery 35–40 miles

Week 46 - Prepping 50–54 miles, long runs 16 and 8 miles

Week 47 - Tapering 24–32 miles

Week 48 - **Race 100 Miles!**

Week 1
Building / Total Miles: 39–50, Long runs 10–12 and 7–9 miles

When you take on the goal of training for a 100-mile race, it helps to break up the process into manageable sections. (This lesson will apply later when you run the 100-mile race, see Race Day Preparations: Ready? Set?, page 199) As you train, think about each day, week or building phase. As these pile on top of each other, you will find yourself trained and ready to run 100 miles. Remember, you are not starting from scratch; you have trained your system before. As you move into these longer miles and mental preparations for your longest race distance yet, hold on to the base reason of why (Chapter One, "What is motivating you to run an Ultra?" page 9). Why do you want to do this? Believe me, you will have to remind yourself now and again.

MONDAY: 4-6 miles easy. Core strength exercises.	Week 1, day 1 of a 48-week training program! This is significant and impressive. To commit to and train for a 100-mile race is a huge life accomplishment in itself. Take note of the fire, excitement and commitment you feel on this day and try to carry it through the entire 12 months.
TUESDAY: 15 min warm up. PYRAMID workout: 2, 4, 6, 4, 2 with equal recovery. 15 min cool down. ~7-10 miles.	These are relatively short intervals with a lot of recovery, so work at a challenging pace, one that you can sustain, but you feel like you are pushing to achieve. Keep moving at a recovery jog pace in between the efforts. This work is to help you test different leg speed and workout paces. Paying attention here will help you perform better in future workouts. (see Run Workout Descriptions, Pyramid, page 48)
WEDNESDAY: 6 miles easy.	
THURSDAY: Rest OR active recovery/ 35-45 min cardio.	See Run Workout Descriptions, Cardio, page 48.
FRIDAY: 5-7 miles steady. Core strength exercises.	While this mileage is not high compared to what you will be running, these next three days of back-to-back-to-back runs can feel like a big start to a first week if you are just coming back to training. Be easy on yourself and ease in.
SATURDAY: 10-12-mile long run.	Check out an old favorite route, see where your pacing is at compared to previous times and take note for future reference. Set a standard for your sleep habits by resting well and recovering between runs.
SUNDAY: 7-9 miles steady.	

Week 2
Building / Total Miles: 41–50, Long runs 12–14 and 10–12 miles

This week is about being consistent with your daily workouts and looking forward to more mileage over the weekend. You continue to build more miles next week, so be sure to finish this one feeling strong and ready for more!

MONDAY: Rest.	Stretching and foam rolling will be helpful! You can add some core strength exercises today, but nothing too intense.
TUESDAY: 5 miles steady. Core strength exercises.	To ready yourself for tomorrow's workout, throw a few 30-second surges into the later half of your run. Three to four will feel good and leave you ready for a hard effort tomorrow. Recover at your easy pace in-between.
WEDNESDAY: 15 min warm up. REVERSE LADDER 10, 8, 6, 3, 2, 1 with half time recovery. 15 min cool down. ~8–11 miles.	Normally you would climb a ladder (see Run Workout Descriptions, LADDER, page 48), but with this workout the longest repeat is first and the times successively decrease. Start with a pace that you can sustain and aim to finish the last few with more intensity. Recovery jog in-between the efforts. Note that the recovery time is half of the interval time.
THURSDAY: Rest/active recovery. 45 min cardio.	An extra rest day this week, which means more mileage on the days you do run.
FRIDAY: 6–8 miles easy. Core strength exercises.	Be sure to mix up your core strength routine. Try different exercises to work your whole body.
SATURDAY: 12–14-mile long run.	Long run of the week.
SUNDAY: 10–12-mile long run.	Follow yesterday's long run with another today to top off your weekly mileage.

Week 3
Building / Total Miles: 50–58, Long runs 18 and 14 miles

This will be a pretty solid mileage week, with a tough speed workout on hump day. Learn to love this workout; it is a super beneficial one for pacing and training your threshold. It is hard and it will challenge your cardio system, but in the 60–90 minutes that it takes you to complete it, you will feel like you got more out of the time than a 3–4 hour easy run. And recovery comes next week, so you can totally do this.

MONDAY: 45 min cardio. Core strength exercises.	If it makes sense to switch Monday and Tuesday, that is an option.
TUESDAY: 5–8 miles easy.	Use these miles to get your legs back under you for tomorrow's speed workout.
WEDNESDAY: 15–20 min warm up. HILL 5 x 5 minutes with 1-minute recovery. 15 min cool down. ~7-10 miles.	You have seen this workout in the 50k and 50M training plans (if not see Run Workout Descriptions, 5-min repeats, page 49). Now, take this speed session to a hill. Having a consistent runnable hill might be the best for this one (even if your race course requires you to power hike). Working on your running stamina on hills is a great way to build confidence and strength. This will be tough with only 1-minute recovery periods. Plan a little reward for getting through this one!
THURSDAY: 6–8 miles easy. Core strength exercises.	Definitely move today. These miles might feel a little funny, and your legs may be heavy. Be sure to keep the miles easy and shake out yesterday's workout. Take note of how your body is feeling for the core strength exercise workout; if you are okay, work on legs a bit more than normal. You have a rest day tomorrow.
FRIDAY: Rest.	Prepare for some LONG miles this weekend!!!
SATURDAY: 18 miles.	This is a jump in your long run mileage followed by another big day tomorrow. Listen to your body and choose terrain that you are ready for. Prepare for more time on the trails and plan for the necessary recovery nutrition so that you are ready for more tomorrow!
SUNDAY: 14-mile long run.	You can do it—the legs might be a little tired and/or stiff from this week and yesterday's effort. Take your time to warm up, fuel, hydrate and move through these fun miles. And keep in mind you are moving into a recovery week!

Week 4
Recovery / Total Miles: 19–28

You've definitely earned this one! Hopefully you feel ready to chill a bit. Write brief notes of how you feel each day. (If you are not already using the Athlete Log, EXTRA PIECES page 214, start now!) Are you tired early in the week? Does that improve by Wednesday or Thursday? How about your appetite? You may be super hungry even by mid-week. Your body is likely making up for the potential caloric deficit accumulated last week. Your sleep and caloric requirements will continue to increase as we get into longer training miles. It is good to pay attention now so that you are more aware later.

MONDAY: Rest.	Stretch and foam roll, but do not think about running at all if you can help it. :)
TUESDAY: 3–5 miles easy. Core strength exercises.	
WEDNESDAY: 5 miles easy or 45–60 min cardio.	
THURSDAY: Rest from running. Core strength exercises.	Hopefully your body is starting to feel recovered and you can put in a good effort on the core strength exercises workout today.
FRIDAY: 5–8 miles as you feel.	
SATURDAY: 6–10 miles easy.	
SUNDAY: Rest.	

Week 5

Building (Hills) / Total Miles: 51–59, Long runs 10 and 18 miles

This is your first focused building block. Your weekly workout for the next three weeks requires you to find a variety of different running grades. Ideally you will work on terrain that is similar to your racecourse, but there are some workouts that I encourage you to find a runnable grade (even if your race course is steeper or flatter). It is good to gain strength and confidence from running uphill.

MONDAY: 5 miles steady. Core strength exercises.	Think about intensifying your core strength exercises routine in the early part of each building phase when you have more time. As the weekly mileages increase, there will be less time for these exercises. Lead off each phase with solid core strength exercise workouts two-three times a week. On week 3 of each build phase you might only get in one-two core strength workouts.
TUESDAY: 5–8 miles easy.	Keep in mind you have a tough workout tomorrow!
WEDNESDAY: 15–20 min warm up. HILL workout: 1) 3 x 6–8 minutes uphill power hiking w/3 min recovery between. 2) 10 min easy run. 3) 5 x 30 second uphill surge with 60–90 seconds recovery. 15 min cool down. ~7–10 miles.	There are three pieces to this workout besides the WU & CD. 1) Find a steep grade that requires you to power hike at a sustainable pace. 2) Run easy for about 10 minutes. 3) Find a grade that you can run, but gets your attention. You want to be all out on these 30-second repeats and fully recover in-between (you can take more recovery time than allotted if you need). Hopefully you can run without interruptions. Make it happen!
THURSDAY: Rest from running. Core strength exercises.	You can throw in non-weight bearing cardio to warm up for your core strength exercises workout (20–45 minutes). Pay attention to your legs after the hill session yesterday. Shoot for 45 minutes–1 hour and hit the whole body, all muscle groups. Just be careful not to tweak or aggravate anything that might be tender from your pace yesterday.
FRIDAY: 6–8 miles easy.	This weekend (Friday–Sunday), keep in mind that you are building into your longest mileage day.
SATURDAY: 10 miles steady.	
SUNDAY: 18-mile long run.	Okay. You might be tired. It's been a tough week. You've got a day off from running tomorrow (don't forget core strength exercises though!). Do not do anything that is going to injure you. When you start a run tired, it is good to use these miles for mental training. Take your time to warm up and feel your body kick into action. It may take 20 minutes to an hour before you feel like you are really moving. Focus on hydration and nutrition as aids to get you through this. Taking in a few more calories than you are used to might make this a little easier. Definitely recover well afterward.

Week 6

Building (Hills) / Total Miles: 50-61, Long run 18-20 and 6-8 miles

In addition to your hilly workouts, add at least one other run where you are working on your hill running and power hiking. Plan ahead for good, hilly locations and possible travel time if necessary.

MONDAY: No run. Core strength exercises.	Core strength exercises are your only workout today. I hope it is a good one for you! If you feel like you need a complete rest day, then take today off and move the core strength exercises workout to tomorrow in addition to the miles. Sometimes a full rest day can do wonders.
TUESDAY: 6-8 miles easy.	
WEDNESDAY: 15 min warm up. HILL 5-6 x 5 min with 1 min recovery. 15-20 min cool down. ~7-10 miles.	Back to the hills for this workout! Find that steady, strong pace that you can sustain through all of the repeats. Be sure to recover well after this! Hydrate, eat, sleep!
THURSDAY: 8-10 miles steady.	Mid-week long run. This might be a little tough after yesterday's workout.
FRIDAY: 5 miles easy. Core strength exercises.	
SATURDAY: 18-20-mile long run.	Plan this run to be similar to your racecourse if possible. You should work your pace on the hills a bit. See how your strength feels relative to the workout earlier in the week.
SUNDAY: 6-8-mile run.	Shake out run to wrap up the week.

Week 7
Building (Hills) / Total Miles: 56–63

This is your last building week of this first hill phase! Nice work! Keep the momentum going through the week and look forward to a recovery week!

MONDAY: Rest.	Finally a full rest day!
TUESDAY: 9-mile run. Warm up for the first 2–3 miles. Keep the middle 3 miles steady. Cool down the last 3 miles.	This is a big run for your first run of the week. It falls this way so that you can get in two good efforts during the week in addition to the longer mileage runs this weekend. Really warm up and cool down at a comfortable pace. Push the middle 3–4 miles so that you feel your effort (aka tempo). These middle miles are your speed miles this week.
WEDNESDAY: 5 miles steady. Core strength exercises.	You have core strength exercises on either side of your hill workout this week, so think about which day makes the most sense to put some emphasis on your legs, or if you want to work full body both days.
THURSDAY: 15–20 min warm up. HILL Workout: 1) 4 x 6 min with 3 min recovery. 2) 5 min easy. 3) 3 x 2 min with 1 min recovery. 4) 5 min easy. 5) 3 x 30 seconds with full recovery (90 seconds). 15 min cool down. ~8-11 miles.	Adding another segment to this hill workout (same as week 5). Remember this is on a runnable grade to build hill running strength and confidence. Continue to increase your pace as you move through the stages. For the second stage, 3 x 2 minutes, try to pick up the pace compared to what you were doing the 6-minute intervals. Increase the pace/effort again for the final 30-second repeats—really push.
FRIDAY: 5 miles easy. Core strength exercises.	
SATURDAY: 20–22-mile long run.	You should be feeling the workouts from this week in your legs. These two long back-to-back runs are the bulk of this week's mileage. Try to keep the middle 5–8 miles of today at good up-tempo pace! Opting for a course with a good elevation profile (mimics your race course) is always something to consider.
SUNDAY: 9–11-mile run.	You have a full rest day tomorrow and you are going into a recovery week! Make these miles count.

Week 8
Recovery / Total Miles: 24–29

Move your body this week, recover from your hill phase, but also check out from the rigors of your training. Use the extra time to get to other projects that had to be countered with your increase in training. Share a smoothie or meal with a friend or family member that you need to catch up with. The training will be back in your face next week; enjoy a physical and mental break this week.

MONDAY: Rest.	A full rest day … Ahhhhh … Enjoy it! Take a mental break from your training plan and goals this week. Just move and enjoy!
TUESDAY: 5 miles easy. Core strength exercises.	
WEDNESDAY: 45–60 min cardio.	
THURSDAY: 8 miles easy.	How do your legs feel today compared to Tuesday's miles?
FRIDAY: Core strength exercises. Rest from running.	You can swap Friday's and Sunday's workouts.
SATURDAY: 5–6 miles easy.	
SUNDAY: 6–10 miles as you feel.	

Week 9
Building (Speed) / Total Miles: 56–66, Long runs 18 and 10–14 miles

Hopefully you come to this first week of the speed phase recharged and excited. Look forward to discovering different terrain the next three weeks for your speed workouts, compared to the hills you discovered in the last phase. Also keep in mind that your weekly mileage is really starting to build. Take note that you have about 60 miles in the first week of this building phase and we are building you to 75 by the end of week 11. Do the appropriate mental and physical preparations to be ready for and enjoy this big block.

MONDAY: 5–6 miles steady.	If you did not do core strength exercises yesterday, you could add a third core strength exercises day to this week if you are feeling ready. Just keep in mind that you have a speed workout tomorrow, so do not put too much emphasis on your legs.
TUESDAY: 15–20 min warm up. PYRAMID SPEED workout: 1, 2, 3, 4, 3, 2, 1 with equal recovery. 15 min cool down. ~7–10 miles.	During your warm up, do not forget to include a few strides to pick up the pace and ready you for the workout. Mellow terrain without interruptions is best for your speed workouts so that you can work on turnover. Make these intervals a little quicker than normal, especially the 1- and 2-minute ones. Run smart and use good form!
WEDNESDAY: 6 miles easy. Core strength exercises.	
THURSDAY: 10–12-mile mid-week long run.	
FRIDAY: Rest from running. Core strength exercises.	
SATURDAY: 18-mile long run.	Just a reminder; use this long run to mimic your racecourse terrain. If you need to work on power hiking or speedy descending, today is the day!
SUNDAY: 10–14-mile long run as you feel.	Run comfortably on terrain that speaks to you today. If the racecourse-type terrain sounds appealing, great. If getting out on a run with a group and losing yourself in conversation to cover the miles sounds better, go for that.

Week 10
Building (Speed) / Total Miles: 68–72, Long runs 20 and 15 miles

If you decided to race week 15 and/or week 30, it is time to start thinking about and preparing for those events (Race Day Preparations: Ready? Set?, page 199). If you have opted to train through one or both of those weeks, be sure to keep the long term goal in mind, the excitement for your 100 miler, present.

MONDAY: 5–6 miles easy. Core strength exercises.	Be careful on the core strength exercises as you are coming off of a high mileage weekend.
TUESDAY: 8 miles steady.	
WEDNESDAY: 15–20 min warm up. 5–6 x 5 min with 1 min recovery. 15 min cool down. ~7-10 miles.	This workout has been a constant in my personal training program for the last three years. Track practice! our small group of friends endearingly calls it. Getting a small group together of similar or varied paces to warm up, execute the workout and cool down together makes this tough workout something you will look forward to during the week.
THURSDAY: 5 miles easy. Core strength exercises.	This is the closest thing you have to a rest day this week. Take it as you need to and if you are feeling like it is too much, this is the day you should rest from running. Do aim to complete the core strength exercises workout though.
FRIDAY: 8 miles steady.	
SATURDAY: 20-mile long run.	Use your weekend long runs to test out race clothing, nutrition and gear. Are there any additional items you need to complete your race kit? Fill in the gaps now or at least make a list (Race Packing List, EXTRA PIECES, page 206) so that you are not stressed as you get closer to your event.
SUNDAY: 15-mile long run.	

Week 11

Building (Speed) / Total Miles: 63–78, Long runs 22–24 and 15–18 miles

This is incredible! Look at what you are accomplishing! These are big miles and tough workouts. The commitment you are showing through three months in is incredible. Celebrate these steps! We still have a ways to go to the big goal, and it is important to recognize the significance of what you are accomplishing along the way.

MONDAY: Rest.	After a tough, full week last week, be sure to truly rest and treat yourself well today. There are plenty of miles coming!
TUESDAY: 6-8 miles easy. Core strength exercises.	
WEDNESDAY: 15–20 min warm up. 6–7 x 5 min with 1 min recovery. 15 min cool down. ~8–11 miles.	Add one more repeat to what you did last week.
THURSDAY: 5-8 miles easy. Core strength exercises.	You can move the core strength exercise workout to tomorrow if that feels better after your speed workout yesterday.
FRIDAY: 7-9 miles. (Middle 3 steady.)	
SATURDAY: 22-24-mile long run.	Do not worry if you are feeling tired or a little slow on these miles over the weekend. You have built up some high-mileage weeks leading up to this point. Do your best and feel good about what you accomplish. Focus on your fueling to help make these miles possible and feel better. Use these efforts to train your mental approach—view these as the later miles of your 100-mile race. How do you want to perform when you are tired?
SUNDAY: 15–18-mile long run.	

Week 12

Recovery / Total Miles: 32–35

Acknowledge that resting this week allows you the time and space to feel recovered and reap the benefits of the high-mileage weeks you have put in to get to this point. Recovery is a very important part to your training.

MONDAY: 4–6 miles easy. OR 45 min cardio.	
TUESDAY: Rest from running. Core strength exercises.	
WEDNESDAY: 5 miles easy.	
THURSDAY: 8 miles easy.	
FRIDAY: 45–60 min cardio. Core strength exercises.	If an extra rest day sounds good and necessary today or Sunday, take one of them completely off. Do not worry about making up the workouts, just rest.
SATURDAY: 10 miles easy.	
SUNDAY: 5–6 miles easy.	

Week 13

Building (Speed) / Total Miles: 59–68

I am pushing you into another speed phase with the potential race on the horizon. Even if you are not racing in a couple of weeks, this is a good time to work on leg turnover. Keeping your legs snappy and responsive to speed (as is possible while training for 100 miles) is the goal. Long-distance miles have the potential to slow down our speed over time. Keeping speed training as a focus early in the program both builds strength and helps us hold on to the bit of speed we can.

MONDAY: 6–8 miles easy. Core strength exercises.	
TUESDAY: 15–20 min warm up. 6–7 x 5 min with 1 min recovery. 15 min cool down. ~8–11 miles.	
WEDNESDAY: 5 miles easy. Core strength exercises.	
THURSDAY: 12-mile mid-week long run.	You can split this into two runs.
FRIDAY: Rest.	You could add a third core strength exercises workout today if you are feeling good! Just be aware of your miles this weekend.
SATURDAY: 18–22-mile long run.	Test your gear and nutrition plan on this run. Plan for a good recovery meal and sleep so that you are ready for tomorrow.
SUNDAY: 10–12-mile long run.	

Week 14

Total Miles: 48–61 / Run 30–35 miles early in week, start 50 km taper by Thursday. OR run 25–30 miles early in the week and start 50M taper by Wednesday.

While you are prepping for your race, keep in mind that you are training through it. I put in my favorite (or not-so favorite) 5-minute repeats session for you early in the week. This should be your last hard paced effort prior to the race. There are always nerves and excitement that build as we get closer to testing our fitness in a race, so tune in to how you expend that energy. There is enough mileage and daily activity to keep the taper tantrums at bay, but you can read about taper tantrums (Train the Brain Chapter Five, Question #4, page 38) for some tips to focus any excess energy that you feel.

MONDAY: 4–6 miles easy. Core strength exercises.	
TUESDAY: 15–20 min warm up. 7–8 x 5 min with 1 min recovery. 15 min cool down. ~9-12 miles.	Run one more repeat than last week.
WEDNESDAY: 10–14-mile mid-week long run.	This is a back-to-back effort having done the speed workout yesterday. Be good to yourself and listen to your body. Decide how many miles to run based on the race you place to run next week (50k or 50M).
THURSDAY: 5 miles easy. Core strength exercises.	
FRIDAY: Rest.	
SATURDAY: 12–14-mile long run.	Keep in mind that you are racing next weekend. You want to run well today, and recover better.
SUNDAY: 8–10-mile long run.	Because you are training through next weekend's race I am still including longer runs this weekend, but I am backing off the mileage a bit so that you have some energy and power for your race.

Week 14 Alternate
Building (Speed) / Total Miles: 64–76, Long runs 25 and 10–13 miles

If you are not racing on week 15, follow week 14 alternate and week 15 alternate. This is the second week of another speed building phase. Take your easy days easy knowing that you have a lot of miles to look forward to later in the week.

MONDAY: 4–6 miles easy.	
TUESDAY: 15–20 min warm up. 7–8 x 5 min with 1 min recovery. 15 min cool down. ~9-12 miles.	Run one more repeat than last week.
WEDNESDAY: 6 miles easy. Core strength exercises.	I would suggest working your leg exercises today (instead of Friday), but don't go overboard with all of the miles you have coming up the next couple of days. In fact, do only body weight leg exercises so that you have some power for your run tomorrow and for the weekend.
THURSDAY: 10–14-mile mid-week long run.	
FRIDAY: Rest from running. Core strength exercises.	Get a full body workout today, but don't over-fatigue yourself. Leave the core workout feeling energized!
SATURDAY: 25-mile long run.	This would be a fun weekend to explore a new trail system with maps and friends. Preparation will be key as there will be more unknowns and you want to ensure you accomplish your mileage goals.
SUNDAY: 10–13-mile long run.	

Week 15
Taper / Total Miles: 58 or 77 miles / 27 miles during week + 50k or 50 M race (part of training)

It is a good idea to re-read the section about Racing to Train (page 229) as you mentally prepare for your event this weekend. Keep your race strategy in mind as well as your big picture goal (100-mile race). Ask yourself what you aim to gain from this weekend's endeavor. And stick to your answer.

MONDAY: 6–8 miles easy. Core strength exercises.	You come into today's run immediately following your weekend mileage. This is all about consistency and training through your upcoming race. You have a little extra time because your mileage requirement is not as high. Take care of any little niggles or pains that might creep in 15 weeks into a 100-mile training program.
TUESDAY: 8 miles easy. Middle 3 miles steady.	Pick up the pace for the middle part of your run. Envision how you want to feel in the later miles of your race this weekend.
WEDNESDAY: 5 miles or 45 minutes cardio. Core strength exercises.	Do not do anything to make you sore or that you cannot recover from for the weekend. The core strength exercises should be body weight only exercises that make you feel nimble, quick and strong.
THURSDAY: Rest.	
FRIDAY: 3 miles easy. 4 x 100 meter strides.	
SATURDAY: 50 km or 50 M race	Stick to your race plan and enjoy the day! Good luck!
SUNDAY: 5 miles or 45 minutes cardio.	Some movement today after the race is a good idea to flush everything through. Non-weight bearing might be your best bet if your muscles are really talking to you (sore).

Week 15 Alternate
Building (Speed) Total Miles: 71–82, Long runs 26–30 and 10–12 miles

With a tough workout early in the week, it is important to rest well in-between so that you can run well over the weekend. Look ahead and plan for the hours necessary to accomplish all of the training this week. Note that next week is a recovery week; there will be more time to catch up on other life details. Plan well so that you can spend your time running this week and keeping up with your priorities. Next week there is a bit more breathing room for life's extras.

MONDAY: 6–8 miles easy. Core strength exercises.	
TUESDAY: 15–20 min warm up. 7–8 x 5 min with 1 min recovery. 15 min cool down. ~9–12 miles.	If you did 8 repeats last week, do 8 again this week. If you haven't hit 8 yet, this is the week to try it! Know that you are stepping into your biggest mileage week, so be aware of this effort and how it may impact your weekend long runs. You have the next couple of days relatively easy. Make sure you take good care to recover so that you can enjoy the weekend back-to-back-to-back!
WEDNESDAY: Rest.	A little (30–45 minutes) non-weight bearing movement cardio or a yoga class could be a good addition to move yesterday's workout through your system.
THURSDAY: 6 miles easy. Core strength exercises.	Go easy on your legs during the core workout today, you are going to need them for the weekend mileage.
FRIDAY: 14-mile long run.	These are great days to take a map and explore or rely on a dependable loop that you repeat multiple times. Find what you are comfortable with and what will make this an enjoyable part of your week's training. If you need to split today's run into two, try for 9–10 in the morning and 4–5 in the evening.
SATURDAY: 26–30-mile long run.	I highly suggest you find a route that intrigues you for this long day. And if you are a social runner, encourage a couple of friends to join you. As an option, your friends can join you for sections of the route. Not everyone wants to run 30 miles on a Saturday, but you might be able to convince a few different people to run shorter sections with you.
SUNDAY: 10–12-mile long run.	This wraps up three long days of running. Take good care! Get good sleep! Expect to be hungry next week!

Week 16
Recovery / Total Miles: 32–35

Whether you raced or continued to build on your mileage, this recovery week is important. Take the time you need to stretch out, foam roll and fuel well. Look over your training log to see how far you have come and how much stronger and ready you are as you work toward your bigger goal. Celebrate a bit! What you have done to this point is significant!

MONDAY: 4–6 miles easy OR 45 min cardio.	I have you moving pretty much every day this week, with much lower mileage so that you can recover. Listen to your body. The goal of this week is to recover. If you feel rest will do you best, then by all means!
TUESDAY: Rest from running. Core strength exercises.	
WEDNESDAY: 5 miles easy.	
THURSDAY: 8 miles easy.	
FRIDAY: 45–60 min cardio. Core strength exercises.	
SATURDAY: 10 miles easy.	Enjoy some mellow terrain and comfortable recovery pace.
SUNDAY: 5–6 miles easy.	If you need an extra rest day, today is your day!

Week 17
Building (Endurance) / Total Miles: 54–67, Long runs 18–22 and 10–12 miles

If you raced week 16, consider easing back in to the miles by sticking to the lower mileage suggestions, especially early in the week.

MONDAY:
6-8 miles easy.
Core strength exercises.

TUESDAY:
15-20 min warm up. PYRAMID (flat ground) 2, 4, 6, 6, 4, 2, 1, 30 sec, with half time recovery. 15 min cool down. ~7-10 miles.

This is your speed workout this week ... there is a hill workout too. Keep a pace you can maintain through each interval with the goal of getting faster for your final rounds. Notes: a) The back-to-back 6-minute intervals will be tough with only 3 minutes recovery. If you need just a little more in-between take 1 more minute (4 total). This should be the only place you add recovery time. b) You do not start with a 30-second and 1-minute repeat but you end with them. Quicken your pace as you return down the ladder, the shorter the time the faster the pace.

WEDNESDAY:
5 miles easy.
Core strength exercises.

THURSDAY:
HILL workout. 20 min warm up. 1) 2 x 8-10 min power hiking with 4 min recovery. 2) 5-10 min jog. 3) 3 x 5 min runnable, steady intensity hill with half time recovery. 4) 10 min jog. 5) 3-5 x 30-45 second uphill running burst with full recovery. 10-15 min cool down. ~8-10 miles.

This is a bit of a tricky hill workout. Tricky because it has three parts requiring two different hill grades. This can be done on a treadmill where you adjust the percentage grade. I always find outdoors much more appealing and inspiring though and often the same hill can offer different grades, as you move up or down, to help you get the job done.

FRIDAY:
Rest.

Move about and stretch and/or foam roll to flush out your week's workouts. Prepare for your weekend runs as well.

SATURDAY:
18-22-mile long run.

SUNDAY:
10-12-mile long run.

Week 18

Building (Endurance) / Total Miles: 67–79, Long runs 13–15 and 22–24 miles

The end of the week has a lot of choices built in for you. Read ahead and think about your options. Write down a plan based on what you want to accomplish and what you think is possible. Try to stick to your initial goals. Be open to adjusting your plan by gauging how you feel as you approach the weekend.

MONDAY: 45 min cardio or rest.	I prefer to have you do a little something the day before your workout so that your legs are ready, but if you need rest after the weekend long runs, opt for rest and run a little longer warm up tomorrow before the workout. You can add core strength today if you are up for it.
TUESDAY: 15–20 min warm up. 6 x 5 min with 1 min recovery. 15 min cool down. ~6-8 miles.	If you rested yesterday, be sure to warm up extra and do at least 4 strides (6 would be better).
WEDNESDAY: 10–12 miles easy ... mid-week long run, easy intensity.	
THURSDAY: 4 miles easy. Core strength exercises.	This is your only scheduled core strength exercise workout this week unless you added another earlier. Focus on core and do not over do it on your legs. You want to have strength for the weekend.
FRIDAY: OPTION 1: 14–16 miles, hilly terrain, work the hills. OPTION 2: 20 minute warm up. 1) 2 x 8–10 min power hiking with 4 min recovery. 2) 5–10 min jog. 3) 3 x 5 min runnable, steady intensity, hill w half time recovery. 4) 10 min jog. 5) 3–5 x 30–45 second uphill running burst with full recovery. 10–15 min cool down. ~9-12 miles.	Your choice. Do you want to run back-to-back-to-back long runs? Or do you want this workout? You can also switch one of today's options to Thursday and take the easier 4 miles today to allow a break before the weekend miles.
SATURDAY: 13–15-mile long run.	You can swap Saturday and Sunday if you prefer to do your longer run on Saturday.
SUNDAY: 22–24-mile long run.	

Week 19

Building (Endurance) / Total Miles: 79–86, Long runs 28–30 and 10–12 miles

You've been going good for a while and this is the last week of this first endurance building phase. Look forward to a recovery week next week! We are getting into your biggest weekly mileage, which means a lot of things: more time on your feet, more energy output, bigger appetite and extra sleep to recover properly. Budget your time wisely, prepare meals and gear bags ahead of time to save you time and ensure good recovery fuel and hydration.

MONDAY: Rest.	Your miles come at the end of the week, so really enjoy this rest day. If you are feeling good and want to run today, swap this rest day with Thursday's workout.
TUESDAY: 8 miles easy. Core strength exercises.	
WEDNESDAY: 15–20 min warm up. 7–8 x 5 min with 1 min recovery. 15 min cool down. ~9–12 miles.	
THURSDAY: 6 miles easy. Core strength exercises.	
FRIDAY: 18-mile hilly long run.	Push the hills! (Power hike, surge a bit, test yourself.)
SATURDAY: 28–30-mile long run.	If you do all of these miles, it is likely you will be over 80 miles for the week. That is okay as long as you are okay. Recovery week starts Monday!
SUNDAY: 10–12-mile long run.	

Week 20
Recovery / Total Miles: 32–35

This is a repeat of week 16. How did you recover last time when I had you moving basically every day? Do you need to throw in more rest to be ready for the next phase? Did you rest too much and want to try to hit the higher end of the suggested mileage this week? Just remember "Rest is Best" on a recovery week.

MONDAY: 4–6 miles easy OR 45 min cardio.	I have you moving pretty much every day this week, with much lower mileage so that you can recover. Listen to your body. The goal of this week is to recover. If you feel rest will do you best, then by all means!
TUESDAY: Rest from running. Core strength exercises.	
WEDNESDAY: 5 miles easy.	
THURSDAY: 8 miles easy.	
FRIDAY: 45–60 min cardio. Core strength exercises.	
SATURDAY: 10 miles easy.	Enjoy mellow terrain and comfortable recovery pace.
SUNDAY: 5–6 miles easy.	If you need an extra rest day, today is your day!

Week 21

Building (Endurance) / Total Miles: 71–79, Long runs 26–28 and 10–12 miles

The miles are really starting to build at this point in addition to your hearty workouts. How are you feeling? Are you excited about the training? Managing to get through? Feeling overwhelmed? Check in with yourself and see what you need to do to stay motivated as we near the mid-way point of the training plan. (Reading Train Your Brain, Chapter 5 might encourage you a bit.)

MONDAY:
8 miles easy.
Core strength exercises

TUESDAY:
SPEED. 15–20 min warm up. PYRAMID workout (mellow, flat terrain) 1, 3, 4, 6, 4, 3, 2, 2, with half time recovery 5-10 min easy jog. 2 x 1 min and 2 x 30 second with full recovery. 15 min cool down. ~8-10 miles.

Again, I'm adding some shorter and hopefully speedier segments, on the tail end of this workout to ensure you are plenty warm and fluid. Note that for the 1-minute and 30-second repeats I want you to take full recovery, which means you need to run those sprints hard and fast and rest/walk/jog recover completely before you start the next. Now that you are endurance trained, which means you are built for miles, these speed bursts will add strength and confidence when done as supplement to your long distances. If your body is overtrained, not warmed up enough and/or specifically trained for speed, it can cause damage. Be careful and attentive!

WEDNESDAY:
5 miles easy.
Core strength exercises.

THURSDAY:
HILL workout. 20 min warm up. 1) 2 x 8-10 min power hiking with 4 minutes downhill jog recovery. 2) 5-10 min jog. 3) 3 x 5 min runnable hill, steady intensity with half time recovery. 4) 10 min jog. 5) 3-5 x 30–45 second uphill running burst with full recovery. 10-15 min cool down. ~8-10 miles.

This is a repeat hill workout from week 17. See if it flows a bit more smoothly this time around.

FRIDAY:
6 miles easy.

SATURDAY:
26–28-mile long run.

SUNDAY:
10–12-mile long run.

Week 22

Building (Endurance) / Total Miles: 76–86, Long runs 28 and 15–18 miles

Time to settle in and feel your body absorb the miles.

MONDAY: Rest.	
TUESDAY: 8 miles easy. Core strength exercises.	
WEDNESDAY: 15–20 min warm up. 7 x 5 min with 1 min recovery. 15 min cool down. ~8-10 miles.	This is a tough workout to add when considering the big miles assigned this week. But it should be short and sweet and take just over an hour to complete.
THURSDAY: 5–8 miles as you feel. Core strength exercises.	
FRIDAY: 12–14-mile long run.	Make it hilly! You know the drill. Make the hills count.
SATURDAY: 28-mile long run.	
SUNDAY: 15–18-mile long run.	

Week 23

Building (Endurance) / Total Miles: 80–90, Long runs 28–30 and 18 miles

Consistency is the name of the game. You are repeating last week but increasing the mileage on some of your longer runs. See how your body handles the miles this week compared to last week. Do you feel the blocks building? Are you recovering faster? Sleeping more soundly? Eating like crazy?

MONDAY: Rest.	You can move this rest day later in the week if you feel like you want to run today. You could swap with either Thursday or Friday.
TUESDAY: 8 miles easy. Core strength exercises.	
WEDNESDAY: 15–20 min warm up. 7–8 x 5 min with 1 min recovery. 15 min cool down. ~9-12 miles.	Do one more repeat than last week.
THURSDAY: 5–8 miles as you feel. Core strength exercises.	I would give your legs a break from too many heavy weights. One-legged body weight squats on a half bosu to work on your balance, golfer swings and warrior 3 with a light dumbbell would all be great lengthening exercises for your legs without over working. You have a lot of miles the next three days!
FRIDAY: 12–14-mile long run.	Make it hilly! You know the drill. Make the hills count.
SATURDAY: 28–30-mile long run.	You might do the same route as last week and add on a few more miles to keep your schedule familiar and your planning easy.
SUNDAY: 18-mile long run.	

Week 24
Recovery / Total Miles: 33–37

You are coming off of a couple of solid training blocks. You have also just finished some of your longest training runs of the plan. Congrats! We are mid-way to your goal!! I encourage you to look ahead and see that the remainder of the plan continues to build. You have a solid base of miles and your body is tuned to receive the coming weeks of training. With that in mind, take a breather this week. Get life in order to be able to accommodate the longer training hours that will be a significant part of the next three months. Build up that mojo and get excited! There is a lot of exploring, both on the trails and within yourself, to come.

MONDAY: Rest.	Listen to your body this week. What I've entered are suggestions, but I would have preferred to leave the entire week blank so that you could fill it in as you go. Sit down before the week starts and lay out what you think will be your ideal and best recovery week. See how it works for you.
TUESDAY: 4–5 miles easy. Core strength exercises.	
WEDNESDAY: 8 miles easy.	
THURSDAY: Rest from running. Core strength exercises.	
FRIDAY: 6–8 miles easy.	
SATURDAY: 10 miles easy.	
SUNDAY: Rest or 5–6 miles easy.	

Week 25
Building (Hills) / Total Miles: 72–80, Long runs 30–34 and 10 miles

This first week of the building phase kicks off with 80 miles and you build from there. Your training base is solid and assuming you are injury free, this mileage is possible. Running this much will take more time over these next three weeks. Set yourself up for success by managing your training time amidst everything else that occupies life and makes you busy. The goal is to maintain running as a healthy, desirable part of your life. Not something that you dread or have to force yourself to do. Time management is a key part of keeping that balance. Also, we are moving back to a hill focus for this block to mix things up and work on strength and confidence.

MONDAY:
8 miles easy.
Core strength exercises.

TUESDAY:
HILL workout. 20 min warm up. 1) 3 x 8–10 min power hiking with 4 min recovery. 2) 5–10 min jog. 3) 2 x 5 min runnable hill at steady intensity with half time recovery. 4) 10 min jog. 5) 3–5 x 30–45 second uphill running burst with full recovery. 10–15 min cool down. ~8–10 miles.

If your racecourse has steeper climbs requiring more power hiking, then do this workout as prescribed. If your course is more runnable switch the 8–10-minute segments for running and power hike the two 5-minute segments. Do the power hiking first.

WEDNESDAY:
6–8 miles easy.
Core strength exercises.

THURSDAY:
Rest OR active recovery/35–45 min cardio.

FRIDAY:
10 miles. Run middle 4 steady.

SATURDAY:
30–34-mile long run.

In addition to hills, this block trains your time on feet (Trick of the Trade, page 30). The goal is to get used to long days running on trails. I encourage you to spend the time running these longer distances so that you go through some of the highs and lows of ultra distance running prior to your race. Figure out how you manage and what your special tricks are to complete these challenging distances.

SUNDAY:
10 miles easy.

Getting back to it the next day might have you cursing me. In the long run, I think that the mental strength you gain from knowing you can run again, even when you are tired, will pay dividends for your 100-mile race.

Week 26
Building (Hills) / Total Miles: 80–88, Long runs 40 and 8–10 miles

With the higher mileage, I am going to keep you at one workout a week and long back-to-back or back-to-back-to-back weekend runs.

MONDAY:
Rest from running.
Core strength exercises.

TUESDAY:
15–20 min warm up.
HILLS: 6–7 x 5 min with 1 min recovery. 15 min cool down. ~7-9 miles.

Find a grade that mimics for racecourse and either power hike or run for the 5-minute intervals.

WEDNESDAY:
8 miles easy.
Core strength exercises.

THURSDAY:
5–7 miles easy.

FRIDAY:
12–14-mile long run.

Fuel well before, during and after all of these runs. Your ability to fuel and recover will keep you going.

SATURDAY:
40-mile long run.

Running with friends for the entire distance or breaking up the milage among a few different running buds will help you enjoy these miles. Also, start to dial in your gear, test sunscreens and skin lubes, anything you think you might help on race day.

SUNDAY:
8–10 miles easy.

Week 27

Building (Hills) / Total Miles: 84–90, Long runs 45 and 8–10 miles

More rest this week, but much longer mileage days when you do run. Please see my note on Friday's run if you are running a race on week 31.

MONDAY: Rest from running. Core strength exercises	
TUESDAY: 12–15 mile hilly long run.	Push the hills similar as you would in a workout.
WEDNESDAY: 5–6 miles easy. Core strength exercises.	
THURSDAY: Rest.	
FRIDAY: 14-mile long run.	If you are racing a 50M or 100km on or around week 31 and you are questioning if you will recover from this weekend's mileage, it is your job to scale it back to a number that is manageable for you. To prepare for your 100-mile race I encourage you to run around 25–30 miles on Saturday and 15–20 either Friday or Sunday and 8–10 the other day (Friday or Sunday).
SATURDAY: 45-mile long run.	This is the longest training run you will do in preparation for your 100-mile race. You may run a race that is longer, but as a solo training run, 45 miles is the longest you will run in a training run.
SUNDAY: 8–10 miles easy.	

Week 28
Recovery / Total Miles: 35–40

I'm curious. How did your last recovery (week 24) go? This week I'm not going to write anything, as I want you to recover as you need for this week. Throw in foam rolling, massage and Epsom salt baths. Whatever it takes to recoup from that last heavy mileage building block. Factor in the next couple of weeks and what your goals are. Will you be racing soon? Are you building through another hefty block? Finally, do not forget your core strength workouts.

MONDAY:	
TUESDAY:	
WEDNESDAY:	
THURSDAY:	
FRIDAY:	
SATURDAY:	
SUNDAY:	

Week 29
Building (Endurance) / Total Miles: 63–82

If you are running a race on week 31, please give this weekend's mileage some thought. You are only two weeks out from a race effort and while you are training through the race, you want to feel good out there. You are more than halfway through the training program and I hope you are learning from your body to know if you should stay on the shorter or longer end of the mileage range.

MONDAY: Rest or 45 min cardio.	The option for cardio is there to prepare you for tomorrow's workout. If you prefer a rest day, you should give yourself a little more warm-up time tomorrow.
TUESDAY: 15–20 min warm up. 6–7 x 5 min with 1 min recovery. 15 min cool down. ~8-10 miles.	It is never a bad idea to do a little extra warm up and two extra strides if your body is not clicking.
WEDNESDAY: 8–10 miles easy. Core strength exercises.	
THURSDAY: 5–10 miles as you feel.	
FRIDAY: 5–10 miles as you feel.	You can add core strength exercises today.
SATURDAY: 25–28-mile long run.	
SUNDAY: 12–14 miles as you feel.	

Week 30
Building (Endurance) / Total Miles: 50–58

This week gears you up for your long race at the end of week 31. There are still some substantial miles to manage this week. Start thinking about the preparations you want to make for your race, how you want to feel on race day and how you plan to recover from each of these workouts so that you have as much in the tank as possible come race day. Keep in mind you are training through this race, as opposed to tapering well and coming into it fine-tuned. You might not feel completely rested and 100 percent on race day. That is okay. Your goal is the 100-miler; this is to prepare you. Know this, and do your best and be happy with your effort.

MONDAY: Rest from running. Core strength exercises.	Do a little cardio (30–45 minutes) to warm up and move your legs to be ready for tomorrow's speedy workout.
TUESDAY: 15–20 min warm up. 1) PYRAMID 2, 4, 6, 4, 2, with half time recovery. 2) 5-10 min jog. 3) 2 x 1 minute, 2 x 30 seconds with full recovery. 15 min cool down. ~7-9 miles.	This is to shock your legs with a speedier pace. All of the miles you have logged recently have the potential to slow down your turn over. It is always good to work on this by tuning the body with some shorter, quicker segments.
WEDNESDAY: 10-14-mile mid-week long run.	You can switch this with tomorrow if you want more recovery after the workout.
THURSDAY: 5 miles easy. Core strength exercises.	
FRIDAY: Rest.	
SATURDAY: 20-mile long run.	The mileage is relative, and now after the weeks you have had, 20 miles should still be an effort, but feel more manageable.
SUNDAY: 8-10-mile run.	

Week 30 Alternate

Building (Endurance) / Total Miles: 83–94, Long runs 35–40 and 8–12 miles

If running a 50-mile or 100-km race does not work in to your schedule, there are still many benefits to gain over these couple of weeks. There are a lot of training hours required to simulate race fatigue and therefore, forced mental training. Learning to manage your body and mind through the tough miles is what this period is about. To hit 90 miles for the week, you will need to run every day. I have two optional "rest from running" days on Monday and Friday for you to implement as you need.

MONDAY: Rest. OR 5 miles easy. Core strength exercises.	Do a little extra cardio (30–45 minutes) as a warm up for your core workout and to move your legs to be ready for tomorrow's workout.
TUESDAY: 15–20 min warm up. 1) PYRAMID 2, 4, 6, 4, 2, with half time recovery. 2) 5-10 min jog. 3) 2 x 1 minute, 2 x 30 seconds with full recovery. 15 min cool down. ~7-9 miles.	This is to gear up your legs a bit with a little speed. All of the miles you have logged recently have the potential to slow down your turn over. It is always good to work on this by tuning the body with some speed.
WEDNESDAY: 10 miles easy.	
THURSDAY: 18-mile mid-week long run.	You can split the mileage into two runs if you need to.
FRIDAY: Rest OR 5 miles easy. Core strength exercises.	Prepare your gear and your mind for the weekend!
SATURDAY: 35–40-mile long run.	
SUNDAY: 8-12-mile long run.	This is to get you out on your feet for a couple of hours when you probably do not want to. Feel what it is like to get going again after a tough run. This is where the back-to-backs can really benefit you. They allow you to recover a bit (assuming you eat and rest well in-between) and show you that you can keep going.

Week 31
Total Miles: 37-43 + Run 50M to 100K Race

With a race at the end of the week, your nerves might intensify. Keep in mind that you are in a heavy training period and might be a little thin on patience with yourself and possibly others. This is also one of your highest mileage training weeks. Do the best you can to train your mind and body for the most challenging aspects of running 100 miles. What comes up for you this week? Where do you resist? Are you reaching your edge? How do you manage the feelings? Tune in to what your mind and body are doing and feeling as you tackle the most taxing part of your training. Keep notes in your running log for future reference (see Althletic Log, page 214).

MONDAY: 6–8 miles easy. Core strength exercises.	Mostly keep moving this week. Don't do anything that will hurt you for your race effort this weekend but keep up the training mileage so that you are training through the race.
TUESDAY: 8 miles, middle 3 steady.	
WEDNESDAY: 10 miles easy. Core strength exercises.	You can split the run into two if that is helpful. 6 miles in the morning, 4 miles in the evening. Do not do anything to make yourself sore in your core strength exercises workout. Think "strength and balance" exercises that will benefit you during the later miles of your race.
THURSDAY: Rest or 45 minutes cardio.	
FRIDAY: 3–5 miles easy. 4 x 100 meter strides.	You might feel a little clunky on these short 3 miles. You haven't run this short in a very long time, your body will likely just start to feel like it is warming up when you reach the end of your run.
SATURDAY: 50 M or 100 KM RACE	Embrace all that comes today. A training race is a tricky piece of this program, mostly mentally. Pay attention to everything you endure today from how you feel physically and mentally to how your gear and nutrition plans perform for you. Write down your thoughts after the race as soon as you can. This is something you will want to read before your 100-mile race, as the lessons learned on this run will benefit you later.
SUNDAY: 90 min–2hr cardio active recovery OR 10–12 miles.	Getting out for another run the day after a race might be impossible with travel or the reality of life after already spending the better part of your weekend at a race. I put the option of 10–12 miles to help you strive to reach 100 miles for the week, but if it is not possible do not sweat it. Racing 50M or 100K is much different than a 45-mile training run and your body will benefit from the effort whether you run 100 miles this week or not.

Week 31 Alternate

Building (Endurance) / Total Miles: 91–100, Long runs 42–45 and 10–12 miles

This is one of your highest mileage weeks of the training program. With that in mind, do the best you can to train your mind and body for the most challenging aspects of running 100 miles. What comes up for you this week? Where do you resist? Are you reaching your edge? How do you manage the feelings? What motivates you? (Running with friends? Rewards?) Tune in to what your mind and body are doing and feeling as you tackle the most taxing part of your training.

MONDAY: Rest.	This is going to be a high mileage week crammed into six days. Utilize this rest day to your advantage.
TUESDAY: 8 miles easy. Core strength exercises.	
WEDNESDAY: 10-mile AM run. Make the middle 5 miles up-tempo. 8-mile PM run. Run up-tempo for 3 x (½ mile, recover 1 mile in-between). 18 miles total.	Today I've split your 18 miles into two runs. On the first, warm up for 2.5 miles, and then run up-tempo for 5 miles and then cool down the final 2.5 miles. In the afternoon or evening warm up for 2 miles, run up-tempo (a little faster than your morning up-tempo pace) for a half mile, recover for 1 mile and repeat three times. Cool down for the final 1.5 miles.
THURSDAY: 8-10 miles easy. Core strength exercises.	Keep in mind that you are in a heavy training period and might be a little thin on patience with yourself and others.
FRIDAY: 5-7 miles easy.	
SATURDAY: 42–45-mile long run.	Try to mimic your racecourse terrain. Also use this run to test out all gear and consumables that you think you want to use in your 100-mile race.
SUNDAY: 10-12-mile long run.	Running on tired legs to remind you that you can.

Week 32

Recovery / Total Miles: 32–37

If you raced last week, aim for the lower end of the mileage suggestion for the week. Please feel free to write your own recovery week schedule. I filled it in with these suggestions on the chance that you do not want to think the week after your race or a 100-mile training week.

MONDAY: Rest.	
TUESDAY: Core strength exercises. AND 4–5 miles easy or 45 min cardio.	
WEDNESDAY: 8 miles easy.	You can switch this with tomorrow if you want more recovery.
THURSDAY: Rest from running. Core strength exercises.	
FRIDAY: 6–8 miles easy.	
SATURDAY: 10 miles easy.	
SUNDAY: Rest. OR 4–6 miles easy.	

Week 33

Recovery / Total Miles: 50–54 miles, Long runs 10–12 and 8 miles

Recovery is the focus of this building block, so we stay with it for four weeks (Weeks 33-36). Your mileage is still building over the first three weeks, but with less intensity on workouts and less overall mileage. Whether you raced or ran the high mileage, it is important to bring your body back around to feeling good. Sleep is the most important piece closely tied with nutrition. You will benefit from midday power naps in addition to your 8-9 hours of sleep a night. You will also benefit from intermittent healthy snacks in addition to your normal meal schedule. Your body is highly receptive right now and you need to do your best to meet its needs.

MONDAY: Rest OR 4–6 miles easy.	Do the opposite of what you did Sunday.
TUESDAY: 8 miles as you feel. Core strength exercises.	No workouts this week, but you can throw in a few up-tempo efforts as you feel today and/or Thursday.
WEDNESDAY: 1 hour cardio or 6 miles steady.	
THURSDAY: 8 miles as you feel. Core strength exercises.	Suggestion: 4–6 x 3 minutes up-tempo efforts mixed within the 8 miles might feel good.
FRIDAY: 6 miles steady.	
SATURDAY: 10–12-mile long run.	
SUNDAY: 8 miles easy.	

Week 34
Recovery / Total Miles: 49–58, Long runs 15–18 and 10 miles

Hopefully your body is coming around and feeling stronger! Now is the time to really feel like the efforts you put in to your training made you feel strong and prepared for your goal race. The more you recover the more the training will take hold in your mind and body. Move well through this block and make sure that you really recover the best you can. If that means backing off the miles a bit then do so! Completing this long recovery after that last block of endurance training is super important to heal and to feeling ready for 100 miles.

MONDAY: Rest from running. Core strength exercises.	Core strength exercises are your only workout today. I hope it is a good one for you! Spend at least 45 minutes working through a full body workout. If you feel like you need a complete rest day, then take today off and move the core strength exercises workout to tomorrow in addition to the miles.
TUESDAY: 6-8 miles easy	
WEDNESDAY: 15 min warm up. HILL 5 x 5 min with 1 min recovery. 15-20 min cool down. ~5-7 miles.	Easing back into a familiar speed workout. I scheduled it to be on a hill/steady incline, but if flat and fast sounds more appealing ... enjoy!
THURSDAY: 8-10 miles steady.	Mid-week long run type effort backed up to yesterday's workout.
FRIDAY: 5 miles easy. Core strength exercises.	
SATURDAY: 15-18-mile long run.	Plan this run to be similar to your racecourse if possible. You should work the hills and see how your strength feels relative to the workout earlier in the week. Stepping back into workouts and long runs after a recovery block is a good way to gauge your body. Note that it might take a couple of workouts to feel fluid again.
SUNDAY: 10-mile run.	

Week 35

Recovery / Total Miles: 52–66, Long runs 18–20 and 10–14 miles

Remember what I said last week!

MONDAY:
6–8 miles easy.

TUESDAY:
Rest from running.
Core strength exercises.

WEDNESDAY:
6–8 miles easy.

THURSDAY:
15 min warm up. 6 x 5 min
with 1 min recovery.
15–20 min cool down.
~6-8 miles.

Test your speed and see if your average pace can be 5–10 seconds faster per mile than you have been working at earlier in the program. The key is that you have to be able to sustain this speedier pace for the entire workout.

FRIDAY:
6–8 miles easy.
Core strength exercises.

SATURDAY:
18–20-mile long run.

SUNDAY:
10–14-mile long run.

Week 36
Recovery / Total Miles: 32–37

As you come to the end of this recovery block and face the lowest mileage week, use these days to prepare for your last big training push. Look ahead at the calendar! You have three steady weeks culminating in a 100-mile week; that is a huge time commitment. What do you need prepare this week for yourself and those around you? How can you stay strong and uninjured through this next training block?

MONDAY: Rest from running. Core strength exercises.	I think you should rest this day after the weekend's mileage and put more effort into your core strength exercises routine. Work on the exercises that are the trickiest for you and bring the most satisfaction after the workout.
TUESDAY: 4–5 miles easy OR 45 minutes cardio.	
WEDNESDAY: 8 miles easy. Core strength exercises.	It is okay to push the core strength exercises this week and even be a little sore even afterwards. As always be careful to avoid any injury!
THURSDAY: Rest.	
FRIDAY: 6–8 miles easy. Core strength exercises.	I'm adding a third day of core strength exercises this week because I want you to put some extra emphasis on building and maintaining all of your stabilizing and supporting muscles.
SATURDAY: 10 miles easy.	
SUNDAY: Rest or 4–6 miles easy.	

Week 37

Building (Endurance) / Total Miles: 86–94, Long runs 30–34 and 12–14 miles

The building block that lies ahead is significant for many reasons. The weeks are big and the time commitment is high. You have done this mileage before, so you know you can manage it. Refer back to your notes during weeks 25, 26 and 27. Is there anything you can learn from that period of similar mileage and apply the lessons here? Keep in mind you are further along in your training plan, with more miles on your legs. Recovery remains crucial.

MONDAY: 8 miles easy. Core strength exercises.	You only have the one workout this week, and the bulk of your training comes over the weekend. Put energy into this core workout while you are still fresh from your recovery block.
TUESDAY: 20 min warm up. HILL 1) 3 x 8–10 min power hiking with 4 min recovery. 2) 5–10 min jog. 3) 2 x 5 min runnable hill, steady intensity with half time recovery. 4) 10 min jog. 5) 3–5 x 30–45 second uphill running burst with full recovery. 10–15 min cool down. ~10-12 miles.	If your racecourse has steeper climbs requiring more power hiking, then do this workout as prescribed. If your course is more runnable and has less climbing, switch the 8–10 minute segments for running and power hike the two 5-minute segments. Do the power hiking first.
WEDNESDAY: 10 miles easy.	
THURSDAY: 6 miles easy. Core strength exercises.	
FRIDAY: 10 miles, run middle 4 steady.	Increase your pace for the middle four miles so that you feel a difference in your pace and effort. This should leave you feeling good and excited for tomorrow's long run.
SATURDAY: 30–34-mile long run.	This is the time to test everything! You want to increase your familiarity with your hydration pack, shorts, pockets, jackets, sunscreen and gloves. Using everything that you might need during your 100-mile race will minimize silly, time-consuming errors. My advice: use these next three weekends to really dial in your system and make notes.
SUNDAY: 12–14 miles easy.	

Week 38
Building (Endurance) / Total Miles: 85–96, Long runs 35 and 20–25 miles

At this point, you are walking a fine line of feeling über fit or over trained. Imagine a sharp ridgeline and you are cruising along the top. You do not want to misstep. This is where all of the awareness you have built comes into play. How do you manage and listen to your body to keep everything in balance? Maintain the ridgeline you've worked so hard for.

MONDAY: Rest from running. Core strength exercises.	You can take a complete rest day and move core strength exercises to Tuesday.
TUESDAY: 6 miles easy.	
WEDNESDAY: 15–20 min warm up. HILLS: 6–7 x 5 min with 1 min recovery. 15 min cool down. ~7–9 miles.	Find a grade that works for your racecourse and either power hike or run it (what do YOU need?) for the 5-minute intervals.
THURSDAY: 5–7 miles easy. Core strength exercises.	
FRIDAY: 12–14-mile long run.	
SATURDAY: 35-mile long run.	Today and tomorrow are your last long back-to-back efforts. These runs allow you to recover in-between, but still show you that you can push through when you are tired. Pretty key lesson for enduring a 100 miler.
SUNDAY: 20–25 mile long run.	Remember you are in control of your mileage and training. Choose mileage and time that you can manage.

Week 39
Building (Endurance) / Total Miles: 82–94, Long runs 35–40 and 8–10 miles

This week you have a longer run on Saturday, but half as many miles on Sunday (compared to last week). The back-to-back allows recovery in-between while still reinforcing your ability to run when the muscles are tired. There is no doubt you will still be tired from last weekend's back-to-back coupled with the miles from the early part of this week. Saturday's long run gets your body ready for a straight through enduring effort. If you have any doubts, look ahead! This is it! This is your final week of hefty mileage. I will keep you consistent with your mileage, but after this weekend the efforts are about dialing in your body to feel strong, recovered and ready.

MONDAY: Rest from running. Core strength exercises.	Look ahead and make a plan for your mileage this week. What is realistic for you to accomplish?
TUESDAY: 8–10 miles easy.	
WEDNESDAY: 12–15-mile hilly long run. Push the hills similar as you would in a workout.	This is your workout of the week. Make the most of the hills. I would guess that you will still be tired from the weekend, so just do your best. And if your best is taking it easier today so that you can get in the long run this weekend, then I totally encourage that!
THURSDAY: 5 miles easy. Core strength exercises.	
FRIDAY: 14-mile long run.	As you total your mileage for the week you are close to hitting 100 miles. If that is a goal for you and your body is strong, add a few miles to these weekend back-to-back runs.
SATURDAY: 35–40-mile long run.	
SUNDAY: 8–10 miles easy.	You are going into a recovery week. If it makes more sense or feels better to rest today and run these miles tomorrow, then make the right decision for your body.

Week 40

Recovery / Total Miles: 35

If you take this whole week off from running you will not regret it. I think it is super important to keep moving and flushing out what you've done up to this point, so find some alternate movements that will keep you happy. A week off now will be very helpful for the mental aspect to build up your enthusiasm for the race and this final block of training. Write your own week as it works best for you. Do some kind of movement close to every day to help your body process and recover from last week's miles.

MONDAY: Rest from everything!	
TUESDAY: 30 min cardio. Core strength exercises.	
WEDNESDAY:	Foam rolling, stretching, yoga ...
THURSDAY:	
FRIDAY:	
SATURDAY:	
SUNDAY:	

Week 41
Building (Speed) / Total Miles: 50–58, Long runs 15–18 and 8 miles

This jumps into a speed training block which will help fine tune your different gears, reduce mileage so that you can recover and keep the workouts fun so you are engaged. If you feel you need one more week to feel more recovered, I suggest following week 46 this week and using the extra time to get back into running (about 45–50 miles). To finish out the calendar bump ahead what I wrote for week 41 to week 42, 42 to 43, 43 to 44, 44 to 45, 45 to 46, then jump back in to 47 as it is. Either plan will work; it is up to you to figure out which is best for you. (You can see this written out on the Distances Summary page 109 and the option Alternative Final Week schedule at the beginning of the 100 Mile Training Plan Section.)

MONDAY: 5–6 miles steady. Core strength exercises.	You have a speed workout tomorrow, so do not put too much emphasis on legs today during the core strength exercises workout.
TUESDAY: 15–20 min warm up. PYRAMID SPEED workout: 1, 2, 3, 4, 3, 2, 1 with equal time recovery. 15 min cool down. ~7-9 miles.	Running on mellow, less technical terrain without interruptions is best for this speed workout. I want you to work on turnover. Make these intervals a little quicker than normal, especially the 1- and 2-minute ones. Run smart and use good form!
WEDNESDAY: 6 miles easy. Core strength exercises.	
THURSDAY: 10–12-mile mid-week long run.	
FRIDAY: Rest from running. Core strength exercises.	
SATURDAY: 15–18-mile long run.	While out on a long run, it is still a good idea to find a quicker pace now and again when the terrain encourages or you feel a surge. Let your body stay familiar with jumping between paces.
SUNDAY: 8-mile long run.	

Week 42

Building (Speed) / Total Miles: 61–70, Long runs 18–22 and 10–12 miles

The 5-minute repeats workout is back this week! Love to hate it, hate to love it. It's awesome and you know it will do wonders as you recover from it. Work on turnover a couple of times this week in addition to Wednesday's workout. Your legs are heavy with lots of miles, it is time to get them thinking about that efficient turnover again and the quicker pace that you know you are capable of.

MONDAY:
5–6 miles easy.
Core strength exercises.

TUESDAY:
8 miles steady.

WEDNESDAY:
15–20 min warm up. 5–6 x 5 min with 1 min recovery. 15 min cool down.
~7–9 miles.

With less overall mileage for the week than you have come accustomed to, see if you can speed up your average pace. This should be a tough workout, but you should recover from it quickly.

THURSDAY:
5 miles easy.
Core strength exercises.

This is the closest thing you have to a rest day this week. Take it as you need to and if you are feeling like the mileage this week is too much, this is the day you should rest from running. Do aim to complete the core strength exercises workout though.

FRIDAY:
8 miles steady.

SATURDAY:
18–22-mile long run.

SUNDAY:
10–12-mile long run.

Week 43

Building (Speed) / Total Miles: 63–75, Long runs 25–28 and 12 miles

It might feel crazy having your last decent length long run this weekend, five weeks out from your 100-mile race. My plan for you is that you are rested and feeling very recovered come race day. In your first 100, I encourage you to go in feeling rested first, strong and fit second. The trickiest part about this is that you may struggle mentally with confidence in your training. It is easy to doubt your fitness and preparedness as you get further away from your last long effort run. Believe me, I have been there. I have learned over the years of racing that my best performances are when I am the most rested and even feel a bit undertrained. It is my belief that one run too many (overtrained) is 100 times worse than 10 runs too few (rested).

MONDAY: Rest.	After a tough full week last week, be sure to truly rest and treat yourself well today. There are plenty of miles this week!
TUESDAY: 6–8 miles easy. Core strength exercises.	
WEDNESDAY: 15–20 min warm up. 6–7 x 5 min with 1 min recovery. 15 min cool down. ~8-10 miles.	Do one more repeat than last week.
THURSDAY: 5-8 miles easy. Core strength exercises.	You can move the core strength exercises workout to tomorrow if that feels better after your speed workout yesterday.
FRIDAY: 7–9 miles. (Middle 3 steady).	
SATURDAY: 25–28-mile long run.	Vary your pace and vary your terrain.
SUNDAY: 12-mile long run.	Visualize these miles as the later miles of your race.

Week 44
Recovery / Total Miles: 35-40

You can refer back to a favorite recovery week or write your own. You are honing in on the end here. Make the most of your days to do the best for your mind, body and loved ones around you. The next couple of weeks are great because there is more time available to be with people and passions that you have had to counter for a few months. Put some of your newfound energy back into those aspects of your life.

MONDAY:	
TUESDAY:	
WEDNESDAY:	
THURSDAY:	
FRIDAY:	
SATURDAY:	
SUNDAY:	

Week 45

Prepping / Total Miles: 50–54, Long runs 16 and 8 miles

Start thinking about any last-minute items or preparations you need to do for yourself or for your crew. (Read Race Day Preparations: Ready? Set? Chapter Eleven.) Completing those pieces now greatly reduces stress as you move into the final weeks before racing.

MONDAY:
6 miles easy.
Core strength exercises.

TUESDAY:
60–75 minutes cardio.

Put some effort into this cardio workout. Mix it up with a few higher intensity intervals.

WEDNESDAY:
8–10 miles easy.
Core strength exercises.

THURSDAY:
7–9 miles steady.

FRIDAY:
5 miles easy.
Core strength exercises.

Adding another core strength exercise day this week and next are great reminders to your body of the importance of keeping everything strong and ready to support you during your upcoming effort. You do not have to lift heavy weights to get a great workout. Focus on balance and stabilizing muscles.

SATURDAY:
16-mile long run.

SUNDAY:
8 miles easy.

Week 46
Prepping / Total Miles: 40–46, Long runs 12–14 and 8 miles

If you followed the original layout, then this is your last week of notable mileage. This should leave you feeling great, rested and the miles should be totally manageable. Rest and reset the mental psyche so that this 100 miler is fun! You've been through it with your training, had the highs and some lows, but it seems like the timing is perfect. Now you walk the line of über fit and overdone. Let's keep you on the über fit side by really resting and letting the training set into your body. Recharge and get psyched.

If you opted to use this week as an additional recovery (for week 41), then you are building back into some mileage that will be helpful leading into the speed phase that lies ahead.

MONDAY: Rest from running. Core strength exercises.	
TUESDAY: 8–10 miles easy.	Keeping you consistent and moving each day. These miles should feel comfortable and you should feel strong.
WEDNESDAY: 7–9 miles steady. Core strength exercises.	
THURSDAY: 60–75 minutes cardio.	Put some effort into this cardio workout. Mix it up with a few higher intensity intervals.
FRIDAY: 5 miles easy. Core strength exercises.	You are not running as much mileage and it is a good idea to keep focus on the core stabilizing muscles so that they are feeling strong going into your race.
SATURDAY: 12–14-mile long run.	Celebrate this run! This is your last long effort till race day. Be excited for it and really think about how you want to feel on race day. What do you notice in your body today that you need to get into final order for your event in two weeks? What do you need to do for yourself and those helping you to feel the most prepared?
SUNDAY: 8 miles easy.	

Week 47
Tapering / Total Miles: 24–32

Here is a key point to remember, something I have heard from countless mentors along the way: *There is nothing you can do in your training in the final two weeks that will benefit you on race day.* The idea being that the training effect takes 2 weeks, so the benefits will come after your race. You can, however, hurt yourself doing too much and not being able to recover in time. Take these two weeks to listen to your body, to fuel appropriately and be aware that you are still recovering. With the lower output, recognize that you are not burning as many calories on a daily basis as you were. Adjust your intake as necessary.

MONDAY: 3–5 miles steady. Core strength exercises.	From here on out do not do any core strength exercises that leave you sore. It is time to really start to feel good in everything you do.
TUESDAY: 15 min warm up. 4–5 x 5 min with 1 min recovery. 15 min cool down. ~5-7 miles.	
WEDNESDAY: 3–5 miles easy. Core strength exercises.	
THURSDAY: Rest.	This is a good time to read through your post 50M or 100K race thoughts. What lessons did you learn on that race that you need to apply for your upcoming 100-miler? If you did not race, refer to weeks 30 and 31 training notes to learn from your high mileage weeks.
FRIDAY: 8–10 mile trail run.	
SATURDAY: 5 miles.	
SUNDAY: Rest.	

Week 48
Race 100 Miles!

Keep calm this week and train your mind. The mental aspect is what is going to get you through. These final days before the race, when you are feeling antsy and would prefer to just be running, use that time to focus your mind and visualize a great run this weekend. The energy will be much better spent training your mind than wasting it on excess movement. Remember there is no training run you can do this week that will make your race better; only rest, sleep and good nutrition/hydration will give you the positive impacts you are looking for.

MONDAY: Rest. You can do some of your favorite core strength exercises, but don't do anything to make you sore or that you cannot recover from.	Two rest days in a row! I've never given you that. You must be getting close to something special.	
TUESDAY: 10 min warm up. 3–5 x 2 min with 1 min jog/recovery. 10 min cool down. ~4-5 miles.	This is to sharpen your mind and your legs. Do not do anything to hurt you. This should leave you feeling pumped!	
WEDNESDAY: 3–5 miles easy.	If your race starts Friday, delete these miles. Rest today and do Friday's mini-run on Thursday.	
THURSDAY: Rest.		
FRIDAY: 3 miles easy. 4 x 100m strides.		
SATURDAY: 100-MILE RACE	How exciting! Race day is here! Please read Chapter Twelve, GO! page 205 for my last little tidbits ... I'm excited for you and more importantly; I hope you are excited for you.	
SUNDAY: CELEBRATE!		

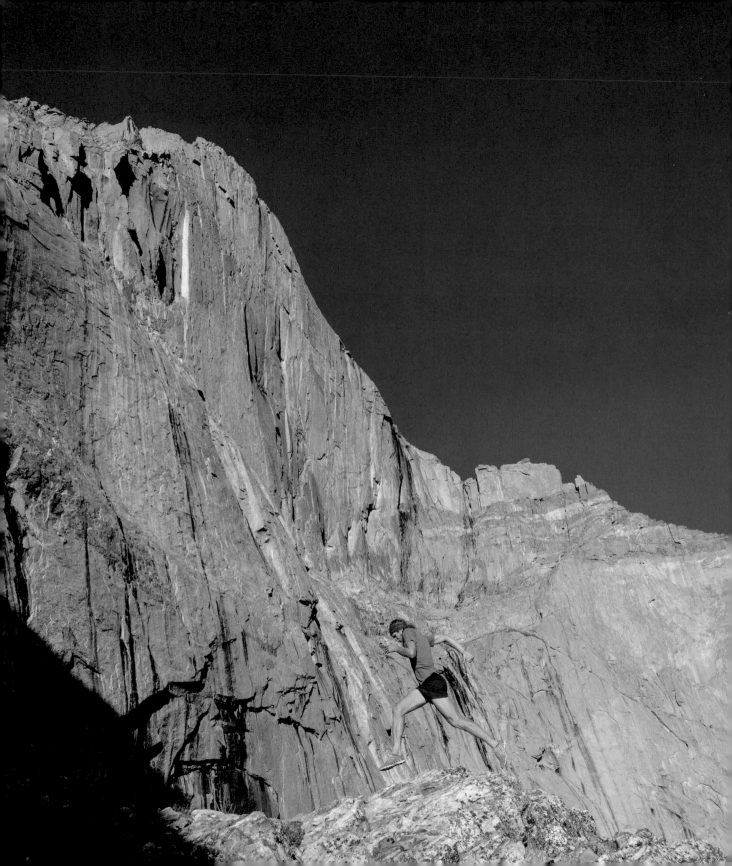

INJURY MANAGEMENT & PREVENTION

Sometimes suddenly (impact), sometimes over time (overuse), injuries creep in and our bodies experience pain while we are running or they stop us from running completely. With rest and treatment, we will return to healthy running. Getting through that injured period can be a tricky game for mind and body.

Prevention comes with maintaining a strong core, body maintenance (foam rolling, nutrition, massage and active isolated stretching) and strategic rest. You will see rest built in to each week and a recovery week at the end of each training block.

Core Strength (see Tricks of the Trade, page 25) to build and maintain strength and flexibility is a huge aid to healthy running. Through your miles you will train the big muscle groups that running depends on, but it is the strength of all the smaller groups that will give you what you need later in the race. Their support lessens the overuse of the main muscles by supporting the joints. Engaging them enables you to utilize the large muscle groups' strength longer.

Recovery (see Tricks of the Trade, page 24) In addition to your nutrition and recover windows, when you finish your run it is essential to focus in on what you need to recover. When it would be easiest to shower and return to your job, kids, computer, etc., give yourself 15 minutes to stretch and/or foam roll while your body is loose and warm from the run. If you can make time, especially after your long runs, soaking in an ice bath or frigid river for 10-15 minutes may aid recovery as well. If you are worried about time, think about avoiding injury. An injury takes weeks or months to heal. Fifteen minutes of care after a run will promote longevity.

Figure Out Your Pain As the miles build, the chances of injury increase. The ultrarunner mentality has an ability to take on too much too fast. It is easy to get caught up in the mileage of a set training plan and of those around you. In some communities, it is easy to be surrounded by people training for long distances and your 20-mile run can feel insignificant in comparison.

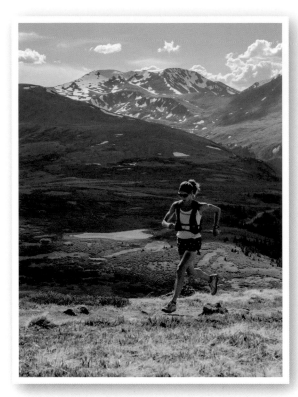

Even if you do everything right with nutrition, strengthening and body maintenance, niggles, pain and injury are possible. As the body adapts to the new workload, you may experience sore and/or tight muscles, tight pulling on your joints and other pains that can limit or prohibit your running stride until you deal with them. As you **identify** your pain and possible injury, ask yourself the following questions:

➜ When does it hurt? Always? Only when running? Before and after running, but not during?

➜ What makes the pain worse?

➜ Where does it hurt? Can I make it hurt by palpating (pressing on) it?

➜ How does the pain present? Sharp? Dull? Ache? Pulling?

➜ What can you do to make it feel better? Stretch? Ice? Heat? Rest?

➜ How many miles are on your shoes? Are you running in the best model for your running form?
(See Gear, page 181 and Tricks of the Trade, page 17)

➜ How are you managing pain? Ibuprofen? Arnica? Natural anti-inflammatory supplements: turmeric and Zyflamend?

FIX IT

Taking an aggressive approach with your treatment by working with health care professionals is the most effective method in my experience. Communicate the answers to the above questions to your **doctor or physical therapist** to help with the diagnosis. Knowing exactly what you are dealing with will allow you to better focus on how to heal. Make sure to work with a professional who understands the runner mindset and body. Find someone who is experienced and sensitive and will educate you how to run/train during these times, not simply tell you to stop running. (Unless of course the injury demands time off from running.)

Other tactics include **massage therapy**, which will help keep muscle fibers aligned. **Acupuncture** keeps the nervous system in check and encourages healing blood flow to problem areas. Strengthening your core, cross-training, examining running form (working with a physical therapist or running coach) and dialing in nutrition all bring understanding of the contributing factors and produce healing results. I choose to invest the time that I would spend running (if I wasn't injured) into actively healing my injury. I also feel it is important to not dwell on the pain or inability to run. Especially when you have a diagnosis and treatment plan, remain positive and focus all energy on the healing process.

With my recent impinged femoral nerve injury, which referred sharp, building pain to my medial knee, I initially dealt with dreadful internal questioning. Did I tear my meniscus? Am I running bone on bone? Is this the injury that is going to take me down for months? I feel very lucky that in 15 years of ultrarunning, the injuries I've sustained are ones I've worked through in four–eight weeks. That said, there is always wonderment if "this is the one" and how will I cope if eight weeks turns into eight months.

Working with my PT, thinking outside the box, charging through my symptoms, pulling out anatomy books and reviewing all possibilities are what helped us reach a working diagnosis. Armed with the pinched femoral nerve diagnosis, I was able to change my mindset and treatment. This incredible shift in my mental view of this injury was a huge adjustment in my treatment and recovery. Now when I run, I think about my hip and visualize that nerve bound up in the joint. I work to keep my feet from reaching forward, and tuck my pelvis to give space to that otherwise limited area. I stop and stretch to allow more space. And wouldn't you know it—the pain in my knee subsides.

Perhaps the hardest part of facing injury is the **mental aspect**. Check the Train your Brain chapter, page 33 for the "what if" questions and specific approaches to mindfully working through injury.

Invincibility is another concern. Running 30 miles Saturday followed by 15 miles on Sunday without soreness Monday might make you feel as though you've broken through a training barrier and your body can handle anything. Then you head out Tuesday to do an easy 5-mile run and pull your hamstring or calf (I've done the latter). It is valuable to respect your training and give thanks to your body for what you have endured. Read through your training log with a keen eye, or have a non-ultrarunner read it and share their thoughts. Is it too much? When did you last recover? Are you unusually irritable? Tired? Is your appetite out of control? Answering these questions will keep you tuned in to your training and recovery and allow you to give yourself extra rest when necessary and avoid injury and/or burnout/overtraining syndrome.

Burnout can be caused by many factors. Namely, overloading the system with physical and emotional stress can tap our system and leave us lacking motivation. Overtraining is the most likely cause—too much training without sufficient recovery. Burning the candle at both ends (physically and emotionally) wears us out and our body will try to communicate the need to recover and find balance. Lacking motivation, always feeling tired, abnormal increase or decrease in appetite and inability to sleep are early symptoms.

Burnout can also be caused by a lack of necessary minerals and vitamins in our system. Some varying theories state that we should be able to consume all important nutrients in our daily diet, but I have found that in heavy training periods, I cannot keep up with my body's demand. Supplementing iron, healthy fats, vitamin D and B are all great additions to help with energy boosts. I feel that the combination of the output necessary for ultra training and the time commitment to ensure all calories, minerals and nutrients are met is immense. (If you have this ability to do this purely through food, I stand in awe!) It is helpful to look into supplements with the guidance of a professional (naturopath or doctor) to keep all systems firing strong. This becomes more imperative if you feel depleted.

Burnout can also be caused by the demands of an ultratraining plan. Adjusting to this new workload, tracking mileage, packing training bags and planning routes all take time. If any of these tasks related to your training become tedious, I encourage you to first acknowledge that this is a common phase of ultratraining and then take a break. Rework the schedule to step away from the plan, rebuild your love and restate your reason for engaging in this goal. Find the basic principles of running that attracted you in the first place. Avoid major burnout by maintaining your psyche. I find running without a watch, meeting up with non-running friends (so that there is no chance of the conversation turning to mileage or splits), cooking involved meals, taking an extra rest day and running new routes all ground me and keep me rejuvenated year after year.

After my share of injuries, I know that pushing through (ignoring the pain) or resting without being proactive to heal does not repair the injury. I have to fix myself by exploring, questioning and implementing. The most important factors are knowledge and time. Figure out what the problem is so that you can treat it effectively. Have the patience to give it the necessary time to heal and be an active participant in your treatment plan. It can be frustrating to be limited by your injury, but if you rush the healing process you will likely prolong your recovery.

A Few Common Runner Injuries

Based on the descriptions below, you may be able to gain understanding of your pain by naming the injury. This will also help you as you work with a medical professional to understand their diagnosis and work on treatment options.

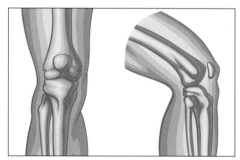

Images provided by Pro-Tex Athletics

1. PATELLOFEMORAL PAIN,[1] ALSO COMMONLY KNOWN AS RUNNER'S KNEE.

Location: Pain is in the front of the knee, around the kneecap, especially below the kneecap.

Symptoms Occur:

➜ When running, walking down stairs or anytime you bend your knee.

➜ After sitting for a while with your knee bent.

➜ Potential for cracking or popping in your knee when moving.

2. IT BAND SYNDROME[2]

Location: Lateral (outside) of the knee (unlike patellofemoral pain on the front of the knee) and sometimes in the hip.

Symptoms Occur:

➜ When running downhill

➜ Increase with running even if you were pain free when you started.

➜ Walking down stairs.

1 Hettrich, C.M. , & Liechti, D. (February 2015). Patellofemoral Pain Syndrome. *American Academy of Orthopaedic Surgeons.* Retrieved from: http://orthoinfo.aaos.org/topic.cfm?topic=A00680

2 Karageanes, S.J. (June 18, 2014). Iliotibial Band Friction Syndrome. *Medscape.* Retrieved from: http://emedicine.medscape.com/article/1250716-overview#showall

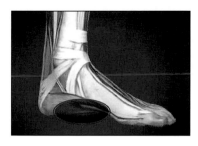

3. PLANTAR FASCIITIS[1]

Location: The band of tissues along the bottom of the foot that support the arch can become inflamed and painful. Especially near the underside of the heel.

Symptoms Occur:

→ In the morning, as you first put your feet on the floor.

→ Increase after running, but not necessarily worse during running.

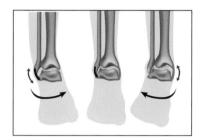

4. SPRAINED ANKLE[2]

Location: Around the ankle joint. Runner is usually aware when a sprain occurs. Can be accompanied with an audible pop and sharp pain after twisting or rolling your ankle.

Symptoms Include:

→ Pain and stiffness in the ankle joint (outside or inside edge depending on rolling).

→ Swelling and bruising around the ankle and into the heel.

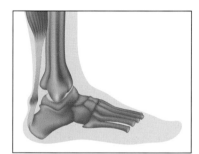

5. ACHILLES TENDINITIS[3]

Location: The Achilles tendon joins your calf muscles to your heel. With repetitive stress can become irritated and inflamed.

Symptoms Occur:

→ In your calf and Achilles tendon.

→ Sometimes at the back of your heel, which can get worse with activity.

→ Increase after running.

→ Along with some swelling of the tendon or a bump at the back of your heel.

1 Kadakia, A.R. (June 2010). Plantar Fasciitis and Bone Spurs. *American Academy of Orthopaedic Surgeons*. Retrieved from: http://orthoinfo.aaos.org/topic.cfm?topic=a00149

2 American Orthopaedic Foot and Ankle Society. (September 2012). Sprained Ankle. *American Academy of Orthopaedic Surgeons*. Retrieved from: http://orthoinfo.aaos.org/topic.cfm?topic=A00150

3 Kadakia, A.R. (June 2010). Achilles Tendinitis. *American Academy of Orthopaedic Surgeons*. Retrieved from: http://orthoinfo.aaos.org/topic.cfm?topic=A00147

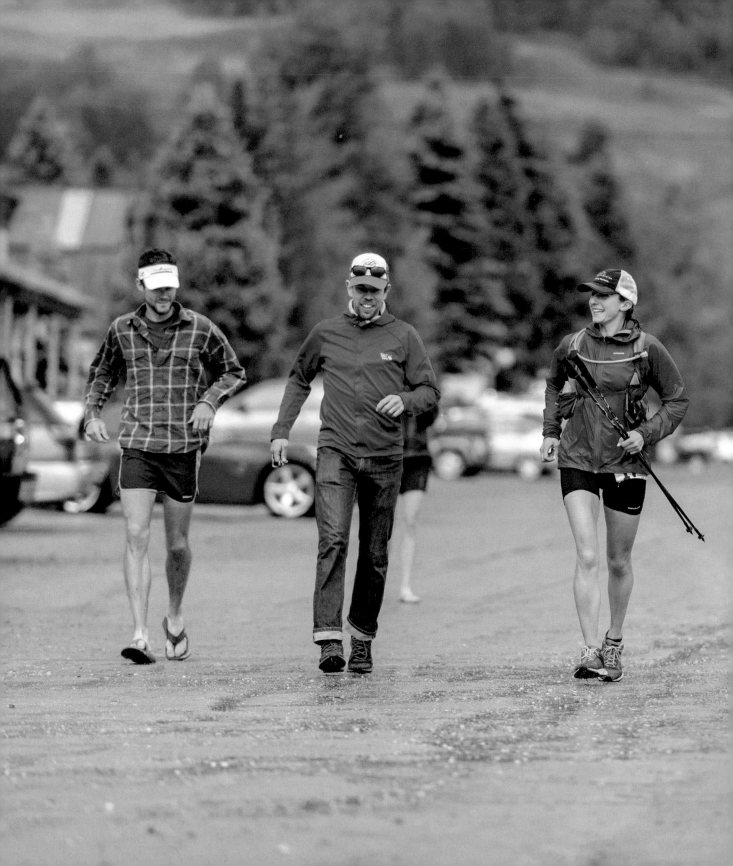

CHAPTER SEVEN

YOUR TEAM

- -

It is important to surround yourself with people that you know you inside and out, and with people you are comfortable with and can trust. This is one of the beautiful life lessons that shines brightly when training for and racing an ultramarathon. The members of your family and social circle, who have always been there through the ups and downs of your life, have the best potential to provide the support, cheers and a kick-in-the-butt to keep you going through your training. Those who have remained through the thick and the thin, and haven't waivered in their support, will make awesome crew members. Think carefully about these people. Will they understand? Can they support this effort? What impact will your running have on their lifestyle? How can you engage them in a way that will interest them?

Those present as your support team will share in your experience for better or worse.

> *It has been said that one can live through the highs and lows of a lifetime in one ultramarathon.*

← "Running with the Boys," Hardrock 2013. More of the story explained on page 189.

- -

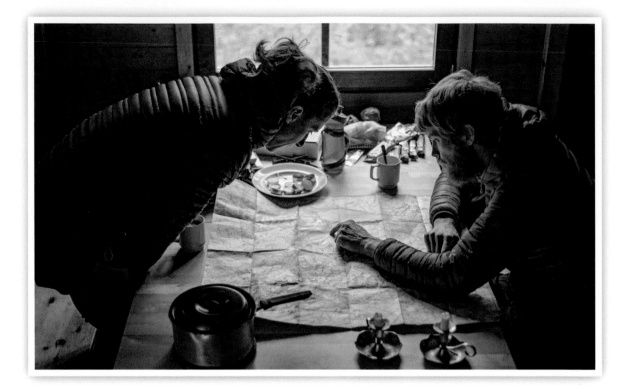

What you need from those closest to you during training:

→ Time. You will need time to train and this will impact those closest to you as your time away is from them.

→ Understanding and flexibility. Adding your training time to the family schedule and/or work is going to be an adjustment for those close to you. Communicate up front about the possible conflicts and plan a rough schedule together.

→ Enthusiasm and support. It's nice to know someone is in your corner when your training is flowing and more so when you are struggling. Engage those that can help you keep balanced through the ebbs and flows.

What you need from your crew during and after the race:

→ A commitment to the travel and rigors of the day spent chasing you around the mountains.

→ Enthusiasm.

→ The ability to notice and act on the little things that will help make your race experience as smooth as possible.

→ A completely selfless attitude from them. Crewing is demanding and requires a personality that is able to set their needs aside for a day+. Be sure to read about crew support, this chapter page 172 and specifically "Prep your crew," page 173.

→ It has been my experience that crewing doesn't stop when the racer finishes the race. The crew is also needed when the run is finished. It is often the simple things, like walking to the car or removing shoes that now seem the most challenging to the finisher. Tending to blistered feet, hydration, recovery drinks, showering and helping the runner find comfort again are all additional crew member functions.

ASKING FOR HELP AND BALANCING THE DEMANDS

The time necessary to train and prepare for your first ultramarathon will require many hours, across long seasons. Additionally, the tasks to prepare for and return from training consume time you might not consider. Time to pack gear, clean muddy shoes, wash clothes and rinse hydration bladders and bottles (do NOT skip this step or you will grow disgusting science projects in your bottles). Time driving to and from trailheads, recovery time, reviewing race websites, buying gear; the total of this time away will impact your lifestyle as well as have an impact on those closest to you.

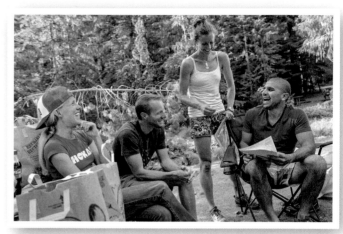

Understanding the demands on your lifestyle will help you realize the impact on those around you. These changes can be an opportunity to grow together and learn from the new experiences. They can also stress relationships negatively. It is

Easy laughs help Darcy and Krissy prepare for the Wonderland Trail FKT 2014.

important to communicate your need for the support and understanding of those closest to you early in the process. By discussing your schedule upfront and checking in on a regular basis, you can create an open line of communication and hopefully have a positive, shared experience.

Suggestions:

1. Share your training calendar and ask for their encouragement to help you execute on your scheduled runs.

2. Do not overwhelm uninterested loved ones with the details of your training; this is the quickest way to lose their support. If they do not run, they likely are not interested in how fast you did your 5-minute repeats. Instead, mention the local park you found on your way home and that you would like to share it with him/her sometime. And then jump in to help prepare dinner.

3. Be creative with ways to engage loved ones in your training.

   a. Finish your run at a park, at the beach or downtown, and meet up for a picnic.

   b. If they might be interested to play coach, ask them to time your intervals. This might mean you run on a track instead of the trails, but it will be worth it.

   c. Challenge her/him to do core strength workouts together. Do not be competitive or try to beat your partner. Work together so that you both get a great workout.

4. Keep a good attitude/demeanor. There will be times when your training is not going well. You will be tired from your long, hard efforts. You will approach "hangry" (hungry and angry) with unfamiliar speed. Be aware of your approach when addressing anyone and do not direct your fatigue on someone else.

5. Be mindful. Do your best to manage your body through the increase of training. Get good rest. Fuel adequately and appropriately. Get the most out of your time training, and make sure to enjoy time spent with your friends and family. Do not arrive tired and hungry, armed with a short fuse. Think before you speak negatively. This mindfulness starts in your training and shines big on race day.

6. Throughout your training and on race day, make it your job to ensure that your crew has the best time possible. During training, communicate your schedule and understand the time impact on your loved ones. Create special adventures to share your training in a way that will appeal to their preferences.

With a crew's help, you will reach past your own limits. You will dig deep and find what it takes to cover this new distance. Their psyche, support and cheers will help motivate you beyond your perceived capability. Knowing they are 'there' for you through training and racing, even when you traverse the trail alone, will bring lightness and a smile.

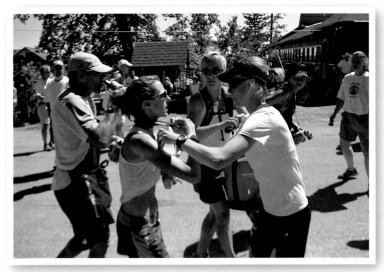

All hands on deck defeat the pity party and push Krissy through the Michigan Bluff Aid Station. Western States 2009.

RACE DAY CREW

If this is your first ultra, it is likely that it will also be your crew's first ultra experience. Be up front with the time commitment required to crew your race. Crewing a 50km race is very different than the extended duration of a 100-mile race. Questions to consider: Will you have to travel? Will you cover expenses? Will your crew person be solo or with multiple supporters? Sharing these important pieces of information and listening to their responses and concerns will allow you to gauge their interest, and together you can make a decision. This does not have to be a serious, fact-driven interchange. In fact, it should be a fun and easy conversation. Keep it light and remember this will be an amazing shared experience.

If you happen to have an experienced ultrarunner in your close social circle that you would like to share your race with, then having them on board could be very helpful. Their personal understanding of ultramarathons, the logistics and the highs and lows a runner may experience will benefit you and your crew. Whether you have an ultrarunner on board or everyone is as green to this as you are, use the following to prepare.

The more informed you are about your event, the easier it will be for your crew.

Participating in over 100 ultra events has meant a number of amazing crews. They work NASCAR pit crew style to move me through aid stations with lightning speed, efficiency and positivity. Imagine the buzzing drills and the quick communication between driver and crew chief: wheels off, wheels on. Then before the fans blink, the car is racing out of the pit and someone stops the watch yelling the time, "18 seconds!" The scene is not quite as loud at a trail-ultra aid station, but similar in productivity when done right. Pockets emptied of garbage, nutrition and hydration replaced, wipe down a sweaty face, spray on sunscreen, give a hug and keep on moving. In 2009, at the Western States 100-mile Endurance Challenge, my team made it their goal to the be the best crew ever.

On race day, in addition to my well-planned crew bags, nerdy spreadsheets and detailed lists, my crew showed up in matching jerseys, armed with special trail treats and the best attitudes a runner could imagine. Amidst the 4 a.m. race chaos, my five amigos hugged me in turn and made sure I had every possible item covered. Devon even rubbed sunscreen on my nose. Charged by their support, I surged up the four-mile climb with a huge smile and a mega-dose of GO power. I felt like I was floating!

As with any ultra, as soon as you feel great, it will change. Fortunately the opposite is also true. When you are at your worst, it will change.

The sun rose and the course dipped the field of runners down in to the scorching canyons. The heat cooked me from the inside out and my stomach rejected anything I consumed. After mile 30, at the Robinson Flat aid station, I did not see my crew again until mile 55, Michigan Bluff. Twenty-five brutal miles, during the heat of the day, caused my efforts to remain cool, calm and collected to fail miserably. I will never forget dragging myself in to the halfway point where I finally saw my crew again. The sun and dry canyon air (imagine a hair dryer blowing down your throat) sucked every ounce of moisture from my body. I was completely defeated by the heat and ready to display the biggest pity party of my life.

Thankfully, this never happened. As soon as I opened my mouth to whine, my voice was muffled in their excited cheers. My eyes took in their broad smiles and bouncing bodies as they pushed me through the aid station. They doused me in ice water and handed me a dripping Popsicle. It was pretty hard to execute that pity party with a brightly colored Popsicle in my mouth. Instead of crumbling, their positivity kept me rolling and I am ever thankful for their energy to help me switch gears and continue on to the finish line of that challenging race.

Prep your crew:

→ Make sure everyone knows the race start time AND your race bib number.

→ Scour and devour the race website. Digest the important information, and share it with each crew person.

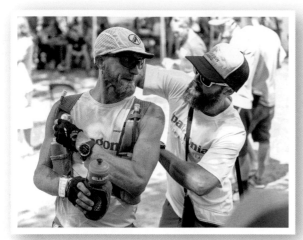

The Bronco Whisperer. George Plomarily resupplies and quiets the bucking Bronco (Jeff Browning).

→ Print off or send links to crew directions and maps.

→ Predict your time splits for the aid stations relevant to your crew so they know when to arrive. Suggest they arrive 30 minutes to one hour before your split time just in case you run faster. See Race Time Sheet, Extra Pieces, page 228.

→ Show them online tracking links (Twitter or on the race website if the race is offering that service) to track your progress. (See Race Time Sheet, Extra Pieces, page 228.)

→ Suggest they bring a book, blanket, chair, warm clothes, sunscreen (depending on the race conditions and time of year), breakfast/lunch/dinner, extra snacks and plenty of water. You want your crew to be prepared and comfortable.

Your crew cannot attend to your needs if they first do not take care of their own.

HELPFUL REFERENCES: (ALL IN EXTRA PIECES)

→ Crew Packing List (page 223)

→ Race Packing List (page 226)

→ Race Timesheet (page 228)

Crew Captain

It may be necessary to designate a crew captain. This depends on the size and dynamic of your group. Having too many people to communicate with and manage can be stressful for you in your preparation and on race day, especially if everyone wants to be in charge. Designating a captain who knows the crewing details can ease stress levels for everyone. This person should know you and your gear the best. They are ideally an organized and detail-oriented person by nature (this is my preference). They are the main person that interacts with you at the aid stations. Other members help retrieve items, calculate splits and manage aid station times, fill bottles, make sandwiches and add fun to the experience. The crew can rotate who is in charge at each aid station, but I recommend keeping your system as simple and succinct as possible.

Attitudes and Interaction

Every race situation is different so it is difficult to make this a turnkey process, but there are basic interactions that can make the crew and runner experience a special one. All crew members need to keep in mind that you are likely running your farthest distance ever. You are amidst a race, where everyone tends to place more self-pressure. It is possible you will mess up your nutrition, the elements will get to you and your suffering could result in a less than ideal attitude.

As the racer, you need to keep in mind that the crew has surrendered their weekend to help you achieve your goal. They are driving through unknown roads to meet you in the middle of seemingly nowhere. They are hauling your gear around, hurrying so they don't miss you and then waiting for long periods of time, hoping you are okay. They are sitting around enduring the elements as well. Make sure they are comfortable and have enough gear, food and water to keep them happy and supplied during the long day of "hurry up and wait."

Greet your crew and volunteers at every aid station with a smile, no matter how great or miserable you feel. Never yell at your crew, period. They do not deserve it and you will hate yourself for it later. Thank them for their help, *every* time you see them. The crew wants to help you. It will be much easier to help you if you are a happy, thankful runner. Plan to have treats and thank you gifts for each crew person ahead of time (you will be too tired to organize this after the race).

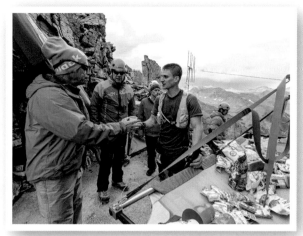

Hardrock 100, Virginius Pass Aid Station at 13,000+ ft fuels runners through the notch.

Aid Station Tips

A dialed crew can be pivotal to running your best race. Over the years, runners have wasted countless minutes and hours in the comfort of aid stations. An understanding crew will help you take care of your needs and move you through without wasting time.

➜ Set a goal of minimal aid station time. You can have one crew member start a watch when you arrive, and make sure that you depart after two minutes or seven minutes, whatever you predetermined.

➜ Set a maximum total time (sum of all aid stations) to spend in aid stations and beat it (assuming you don't completely have to reset after a blow-up) (reference Mid-Race Blow Up, Chapter 5 on pg 40). You are at the race to run. Utilize the aid stations to resupply your hydration and nutrition needs, as well as your psyche and then get back out there.

➜ On the chance that you blow up—be it a massive blister, a major bonk or uncontrollable stomach issues— aid stations are an amazing location to put the wheels back on and finish your race. In this case, forget about the watch and take the time necessary to ensure you are ready to go again.

Regardless of how much time you spend in aid stations, always be grateful to the volunteers and your crew as you pass through. A meaningful "thank you" and a smile will go a long way.

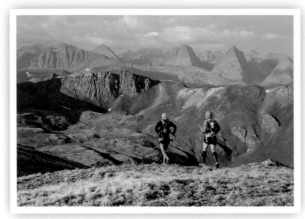

Darcy Piceu and pacer Nettie Pardue head into better weather.

Contingency Plan:
What if we miss each other?

This scenario is miserable for both the crew and the runner, and it does happen. As the runner, you should have a plan for how you will utilize the aid station on the chance that your crew does not make it. Do not waste energy being upset or worried until you need to. If you do not see your crew right away, start your refueling and resupplying process while keeping an eye out for their arrival. As you fill your hydration, ask a volunteer to look around for your crew—give their names. If you are unable to locate your crew before you are ready to leave, let the aid station captain know that you missed your crew along with your name and your bib number and any message you would like relayed to your crew should they show up.

As the crew, check with the aid station captain or timing people to see if your runner has come through when you arrive at the aid station. If you missed your runner, move quickly to the next crewable aid station. Be sure to thank the volunteers for helping you track your runner.

When you do reunite, do not waste time discussing why you missed each other. Keep moving your runner forward. There will be plenty of time to share the crazy stories that happened during the race after you reach the finish line.

A Note to Your Crew

Be aware of the time estimates and goals of your runner, but also take your time and take care of yourself. Review the directions before driving to the next location and/or ask a fellow crew person to help you navigate. There are likely many friendly, veteran crews around you that will be more than happy to assist a newbie. Do not hesitate to engage and ask for help. Allow plenty of time to comfortably set up your vehicle or crewing spot. And be sure to take a moment for yourself. Enjoy the beauty around you.

Before your runner arrives, scope out the aid station setup. Gather an understanding of how the aid station captain is running the show. At some races, there are designated areas for crew and at others you are allowed to accompany your runner at all times. Make sure you are not breaking any rules. It is helpful to acquire the information about the next segment of the course (how far, terrain, elevation, etc.) in case your runner asks.

When your runner arrives at the aid station, it is beneficial for the crew captain to quickly evaluate without asking your runner too many questions. You can tell a lot by watching and observing. Does your runner have a lot of salt marks on their clothing and/or face? Are they glistening or soaked from sweat? Are they dry? Are there a lot of food wrappers in their pack (eating well) or are the gel packets still full? Is their hydration bladder or bottle full (not drinking) or empty (drinking)? Of course all of these observations could be debunked. Your runner may have just filled their bladder, or dumped all of their trash at a previous aid station, or doused themselves at the last creek. But it doesn't hurt to observe rather than overwhelm with rapid-fire questions.

Let your runner talk to you first. They should tell you what they need right away. Make sure you are keeping track of this list and assign one of the crew members to start preparing their requests. Let your runner eyeball and sample from the aid station table, but do not let them linger too long. You can fill (or better, swap out) their hydration pack or bottles while they dine. Offer to sponge them off if it is hot, but do not get their shoes wet. Add sunscreen. Change or add clothing if it is cold. Adjust the runner's kit to accommodate a possible weather transition during the next segment.

As the runner leaves the aid station, make sure you have not forgotten anything they requested. Double check that you have emptied their garbage, that their nutrition and hydration needs are stocked and that they have any gear required for the next section (poles, visor, beanie, jacket, lights, etc.). It is a nice touch to tell the runner how many miles they will run to the next aid station and also how long it will be before you will see them. It is possible that you might not be at the next aid station, but at the following, another five miles down the course.

You will not need to go through each of these steps at every aid station. The race spreadsheet (page 228, prepared by your runner) will let you know the key things to focus on at each stop. During longer races, you will find that aid station stops are minimal during the early race miles and the runner may linger longer later on. Make sure you understand before the race how much time your runner plans to spend in aid stations so that you can scoot them through efficiently or be patient and let them dawdle.

As you prepare to leave, celebrate with the other crew members (or give a hi-five to another crew if you are solo). Your efforts are incredible and you should celebrate your part in helping your runner achieve his or her goal. Clean up your crew spot and leave nothing behind. Thank the aid station captain and any volunteers who were helpful. Take a second to clean yourself from your runner interaction (baby wipes or a washcloth are the crew's most essential piece of gear) and once again take in the scene. There is a lot happening and you might be working on minimal sleep. You do not want to forget the special points of this experience, so make a note to take it all in now and again.

Pacers

Depending on your training partners, finding a pacer can be easy or tricky. This person has the potential to be your late race motivator, on-trail medic and lifetime friend. Sharing trail time is one of the best ways to connect with a fellow human. Typically pacers are only allowed during 100-mile races, but as the sport grows, some 50-mile and 100km races allow pacers in the later miles. A pacer will join you when you are tired and they are fresh, ready to run.

Things to discuss with your pacer before the race:

→ Decide if you want your pacer to run in front of or behind you. Example: When racing, I typically prefer to run in front when I feel good, so I have a better view of the trail. When I am tired or not feeling well, I ask my pacer to run in front, but not too far ahead. You shouldn't have to yell to talk to you pacer.

→ If it is hot, dry and dusty, it is a good idea for the racer to run in front. You both may consider wearing a Buff™ or bandana around your nose and mouth to reduce inhaling too much trail dust.

→ Discuss your preferences on running together. It might be a helpful reminder that this is your race and not their training run. Having a pacer run 200 meters ahead of you because they want to run faster will likely demoralize you rather than help you.

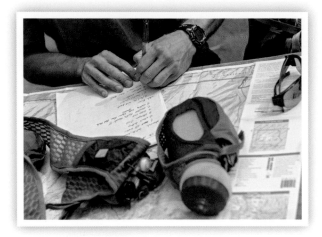

At the race:

→ Your pacer may need to sign in and pick up a pacer bib.

→ Do not allow your pacer to "mule" for you. They cannot break any race rules by carrying your supplies or assisting you physically. (Leadville 100 is one race that allows this.)

→ Your pacer is there to keep you safe.

→ They can remind you to eat and drink and help you move through aid stations quickly.

→ They can chat to keep you awake and entertained.

→ They can offer cheers and support and remind you of your goals.

Drop Bags

Whether you have crew or not, there may be aid stations along the course where your crew is unable to meet you and a drop bag will be your key resource for resupply. The luxury of a crew is that you can basically pack one "drop bag" that they transport to each aid station for you. If you are running the race solo and depending on drop bags along the way, extra planning is required to ensure that you have your necessary items placed strategically.

First, project your aid station arrival times for your ideal race and for your worst-case scenario race. Be sure to note the time-of-day window that relates to each location. For example, if you plan to run the first six miles in 1:15–1:30 and the race starts at 5 a.m., the time-of-day relation is 6:15–6:30 a.m. That might mean that the sun is up, you can ditch your headlamp in a drop bag and pick up an extra water bottle or hydration pack in anticipation of warmer weather. These time-of-day windows will likely expand over the course of your long day. By mile 35 of a 50 miler, the time gap could be 1–3 hours. If you do not have a crew to transport your bag, then you may need to pack duplicate items in separate locations.

Consider: Shoe and/or sock changes. Sunscreen. Lights. Batteries. Clothing options. Energy food resupply. Electrolyte pills. Music. Anti-chaffing balm. Chapstick. Caffeine.

Remember that you are responsible for your drop bags at the end of the race. The race director will transport them to the finish line and you need to collect them before you depart. Please do not put the burden of shipping your stinky shoes or sweaty clothing items on the race committee.

SUMMARY

There are a lot of suggestions of how to create the best crew and tips from personal racing experience. The reality is that it boils down to what works for you and your team. If your entire crew sets out with the same goal of getting you to the finish line and has the best intentions to achieve your magnificent finish, then the experience will be magical. Even when mistakes are made, it is the positive intention that will carry through and create the most meaningful memories.

The final stretch of the Western States 100-mile run ends with a one-mile road section and 300-meter jaunt around the Placerville High School track. For my 2012 finish Ma stood on the infield cheering me on, "Go Krissy Girl!" My crew and pacers matched me stride for stride and I floated on their energy to my new 100-mile PR.

After crossing the finish line, I stood in complete awe of what we accomplished. My knees buckled, and the race director passed me off to the stable support of my crew. Even after the race was finished, I was able to rely on the support of my crew.

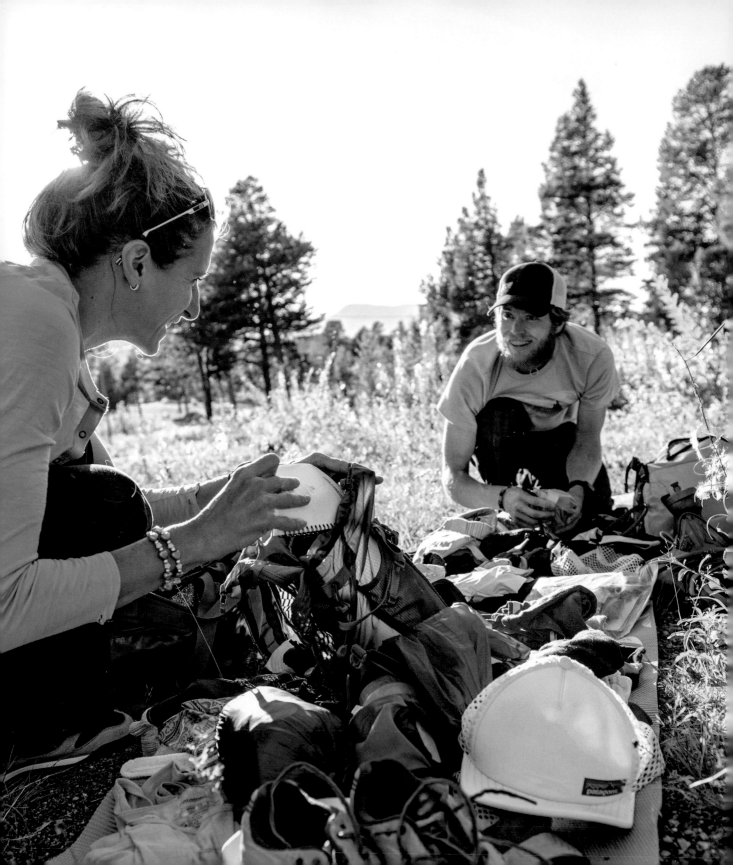

CHAPTER EIGHT

GEAR

- -

As runners, we do not have to worry about bikes, helmets, climbing harnesses, paddles or other extraneous, space-consuming gear (although I love all of these things for cross-training and other forms of playing outside!). Simplicity is the beauty of running; owning a pair of shoes and a sports bra (for some) meets the basic gear requirements. While minimal, we are athletes, and the gear that accompanies any sport can range from basic, to high-end. Super simple to super technical. It is your decision on how much you want to invest in, and geek out on, your gear.

Shoes

Perhaps the most important piece of equipment in the runner's closet is their footwear. How we treat our feet while running, as well as through the rest of the day, will help or hinder our gait, stride and longevity. There are numerous shoe brands and model types available to runners. It is good to keep in mind that just because a specific model works for your friend or one of your running idols, it may not be the best shoe for you. With the many crazes in footwear, from minimal to maximal, abilities to customize with foot beds and tricky lacing techniques, we are lucky to have options. It is important to find the combinations that work for you.

> There were not many "trail running shoes" in 2000. A lot of people ran in low-cut hiking boots or road running shoes. Through design trial and error, growth in the sport and many more brands coming to the trail running market, a lot has evolved in footwear.

← Luke Nelson and Krissy pack gear and food for their seven day adventure on Sweden's Kings trail.

- -

Selling shoes at the Seattle Running Company long before I was a trail runner taught me the basics of our biomechanics. We filmed our customers' running form from four angles while they ran on a treadmill, and then watched the footage for analysis. Our goal was to encourage a neutral stride, where the foot lands on the front part of the heel or mid-foot and rolls thru the mid-foot while the ankle/Achilles remains in close-to-vertical alignment. The pattern continues across the metatarsals and pushes off strongly from the first and second toes. If there were major deviations from this pattern, we would utilize the various footwear technologies to assist the foot and encourage a more neutral stride. From this experience, I encourage you to work with a trained sales person at a specialty run shop. This is a great start to find the perfect pair of shoes for you.

Note, you do not have to choose just one. Having a quiver of shoes is a great idea. Realize there are a variety of terrains on which you will train and finding the shoes that work best for each variation gives your feet and legs alternatives. Just like the terrain trains different body aspects, so too can shoes help your body adjust and strengthen in different ways. Additionally, as your miles increase, it is a good idea to run in different pairs of shoes (even if it is a couple pairs of the same model) so that you do not pound out the cushion and support of one pair. Your body will appreciate the variety.

Socks

For as many pairs of shoes, there are probably three times as many socks to choose from with variety in fabrics, construction and thickness. And just like our biomechanics, our comfort preferences differ, too. When I was racing half marathons and cross-country races, I preferred the thinnest sock I could find. Now with longer trail miles, I prefer cushioning in the heel and toe and a well-fitted instep and ankle. Ankle heights vary depending on preference. I wear low anklets in the summer with a padded cuff (Patagonia Lightweight Merino Run sock) to buffer my Achilles from the heel counter, and a taller, thicker sock in the winter to keep my ankles warm, guarded from crusty snow.

When avoiding wet feet is impossible, either hot, humid conditions or rain and puddles, I prefer a shoe with a mesh upper construction that breathes and drains well. I combine this with a wool blend sock. Wool manages temperature well and expels water relatively quickly and will eventually dry out, depending on the climate.

On even the coldest days I find wearing a single sock layer, preferably wool blend and a taller, thicker ski or snowboard sock does the trick. The key to keeping toes warm is to encourage circulation. Wearing too many layers in your shoes can restrict blood flow even when you are moving. Blocking the wind is also helpful. Wearing a shoe that's upper is a tighter fabric weave or shell fabric will help. And again the final choice varies with the conditions.

In the Tricks of the Trade chapter (page 17), I note 2 Toms Blistershield as my preference to avoid blisters. Other blister avoiding options include skin lubes and different sock fabrics and design options. In writing this section of the book, I had the opportunity to test Injinji toe socks, and while fabric between my toes is very odd to me, I can appreciate the concept. I have friends[1] that swear by Injinjis, as the socks have created ease in their foot care regime. The material between toes means reduced blisters and the independent digit movement gives a more barefoot feel (proprioception).

1   specifically - Jeff Browning, Patagonia Ambassador. 100-mile specialist.

Hydration Packs and/or Bottles

As miles increase and your accessibility to food and water decrease, you will need to look into a pack system that will enable you to carry the gear you need for the long haul. In addition to food and water, you may need to carry lights, gloves, a beanie, a jacket and pants. Maps, a whistle, a first aid kit and an emergency bivy sack may also need to occupy space in your pack. Technology, like your camera, phone and GPS, could potentially add some weight as well. These are all pieces to consider when picking the pack that will support your longer adventures.

Where and how you carry your gear is up to you. The three most common pack options[1] include a backpack or vest style hydration pack with stash pockets on the front and carrying capacity for bigger items on back.[2] A waist pack holsters your goods around your hips making use of pockets and water bottle sleeves. Handheld water bottles with straps to hold them to your palm often have pockets for storing smaller items. Creating combinations of packs and bottles or hydration bladders in packs is the personalization part that helps you dial in your system.

Owning a few options for different length runs and accessible versus inaccessible adventures is also a good idea. The final customization of your hydration kit comes from the ability to cinch and adjust a pack to your frame. I recommend filling the pack to its maximum while at home and making any necessary modifications. (Cutting straps, burning or sewing edges, adding pockets, removing webbing loops.)

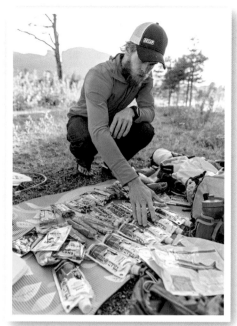

Concentrated Trail Butter calories pair well with quick carb Clif Bloks for varied fueling.

A note for cold weather: Insulating the tube of your hydration bladder becomes necessary in freezing temperatures. The small plastic tube that transports water from your back to your mouth will quickly solidify and make hydration impossible. A couple of tricks include wearing your hydration pack under your jacket to keep it out of the weather and utilizing your body heat to keep the tube warm, or insulating your hydration hose with neoprene or other creative materials.

Clothing

A variety of fabrics, styles and fits create countless options when it comes to getting dressed for your run. Shorts, skirts, capris, tights, loose-fitting pants, wind pants, tanks, t-shirts, long sleeve shirts, long sleeve zip shirts, sports bras, wind shirts, lightweight shells, rain shells, insulating layers, gloves, beanies and many more pieces are available to outfit your run. Having options and putting together the right combinations for the weather is the goal. A favorite saying of mine, from many friends in the outdoor industry and especially the Pacific Northwest, is, *"There is no bad weather, only bad gear."* And I would add that knowing the weather and putting together the right combination of gear will result in a more enjoyable run.

---

1   Some people carry gear in pocketed shorts and women have been known to use their sports bras for easy access.
2   In 2011 I got to design the Ultraspire Omega pack with Bryce Thatcher to accommodate the mandatory gear of the Ultra Trail du Mont Blanc.

Compression

Take it or leave it. I say this because some people believe in using compression while others do not. Some use it while running, others do not. Because my body temperature tends to run hot, any time I've run in compression I have overheated and felt restricted. While I understand the idea of compression increasing circulation and stabilizing muscles during workouts[1] (although the science is showing there is little to no difference in performance with compression compared to without), I feel these potential benefits do not outweigh my discomfort or increased body temperature.

Therefore, I take it for recovery. My body has a tendency to swell after long runs, especially my hands, lower legs and feet. Wearing compression after a long run, post race and especially while traveling helps reduce the uncomfortable edema,[2] accumulation of fluid below the skin, by aiding the circulatory system.

Compression options include calf sleeves, full tights and socks, typically at least knee high. There are a variety of brands offering compression products and most recommend a graduated form, more compression at the ankle progressing to less at the hip. Try a few out and see if you notice any benefits.

Sunglasses

Sunglasses are not only important for shading your eyes from the sun. They are also a key form of eye protection from wind, cold temperatures and in the rare instance when you misjudge, a branch aimed right at your precious eyeball. I once froze my corneas while running a frigid 100km race in Virginia. My vision was blurred for the final 5 hours of the race and for 24 hours after finishing. Clear lenses will be helpful at night for protection from these other elements. Finding the right glass or plastic lens combined with frame to fit comfortably over your nose and ears will make these a key piece of gear. With a variety of styles, frames and materials, what you wear on your face does not have to be purely functional.

Headwear

Style or function, having the right piece of headwear can add huge comfort to the experience. A few varieties to consider include a brimmed hat or visor to keep the sun off, or to block your face if you have to put your head down in a windstorm. A Buff™ will keep hair out of your face, your ears warm or absorb sweat from your brow. A beanie offers an extra layer of warmth, or protects a hairless head from sunburn. A bin full of options will set the stage for accommodating various conditions.

Lights

These may or may not be necessary, depending on your training. At the very least, everyone should own a light source for the winter training months. Those long dark hours can make pre- or post-work runs feel impossible. Having a preferred light will encourage you to get out the door in spite of daylight savings. For those daily runs in the darker hours, I like the Black Diamond Sprinter, which is a great option for a bright and rechargeable light.

---

1 http://www.huffingtonpost.com/2012/05/02/compression-gear-improve-performance_n_1471222.html -- article states that wearing compression during exercise is not as beneficial as projected when worn during exercise. Article goes on to say that worn for recovery it has benefits, mainly from improving circulation. http://running.competitor.com/2013/12/recovery/do-compression-socks-really-work_62611

2 http://en.wikipedia.org/wiki/Edema

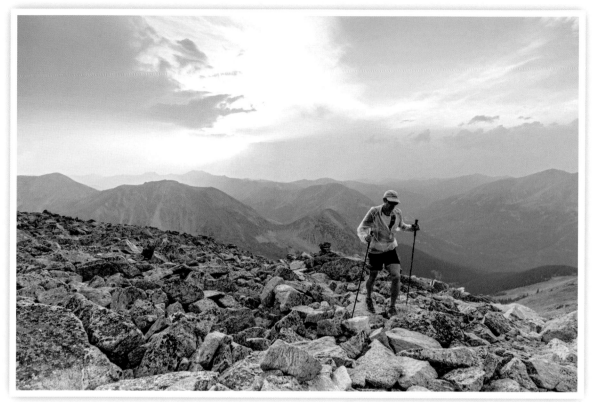

Matt Hart stays steady through Nolan's 14ers.

Headlamps are easy and keep your hands free for eating, adjusting gear or carrying a water bottle. Handheld flashlights are great for directing the light exactly where you need it and to spot off trail sounds that otherwise lurk in the darkness. Adding a light around your waist or holding one in your hand provides a second light trajectory creating better depth of field. I find the waist placement to be most helpful when it is dusty or misty. When wearing a headlamp, the air particulates are illuminated, making it difficult to see. For racing, using a combination of lights to illuminate your path will help not only your vision and forward progress, but it may also help repress the sleep monsters. (See Tricks of the Trade, page 27 for night running tips.)

Trekking Poles

First popular in Europe, these helpful aids started their running boom in the U.S. around 2009. Is using them cheating? Hard to say. They are definitely helpful on long steep climbs and on tricky terrain. I have only used them a handful of times, the most notable of which was my first, the 2009 win and women's course record of Ultra Trail du Mont Blanc. What I noticed was reduced fatigue in my legs, which allowed me to run strong later in the race. Coincidentally, I made the error of having not trained with the poles (in fact I bought the pair I used only two days before the race) and in my aggressive poling to pull myself up the rocky slopes, I fatigued my left anterior deltoid to the point of failure. I couldn't even lift a water bottle to hydrate myself at the end of the race! If you plan to use poles in your race, be sure to train with them.

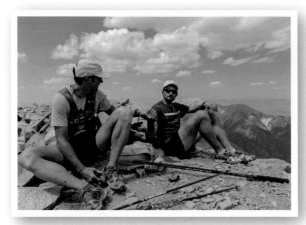
Hours in and hours to go Matt Hart and Jared Campell celebrate another of the Nolan's summits.

Poles tend to throw off my stride and get in the way when running downhill, so I only use them on long, steep ascents to help pull. I typically secure them to my pack or carry them in my hand for descents and more runnable terrain. Many people use poles as extra points of contact for all running terrain. Training with your poles, and becoming familiar with how they aid you will make their use much more efficient. Also, when using poles be very aware of your surroundings and pole placement. Catching your pole on a tight spot between rocks or in-between your legs on a quick descent can result in a fall and possible injury. While in a group, keep your poles close and be careful to keep them out of the way of others.

The current market hosts a limited variety of running pole options. Finding the lightest and most durable option is your first priority. I prefer the Black Diamond Ultra Distance Z-poles, they are collapsible and I can attach them to my hydration pack, while others prefer fixed poles, which minimize weight and moving parts. It is important to note that not all races allow the use of poles for safety and other reasons.

Footing

Seasons and geology are two factors in where you put your feet while trail running. Awareness of your surroundings and the climate will help you adapt as the weather and terrain shifts, whether in your backyard or traveling abroad. In the Shoe section, I talk about owning a quiver of shoes for training your body and for varying terrain. Understanding how different outsole traction patterns and densities of rubber affect whether you stick to a rock or slide will improve your confidence in your footing.

Learn terrain types. Stay light and quick on your feet. Follow behind more confident runners and mimic their foot placement.

Conditions to consider:

- → Mud
- → Clay
- → Tree roots
- → Mossy rocks
- → Sand
- → Desert slabs
- → Hard pack roads

- → Salt flats
- → Ice
- → Snow
- → Steep inclines
- → Steep descents
- → Boulder fields
- → Scree fields

First Aid/Safety Kit

The farther away you are from civilization the more important it is to carry your own medical supplies and to know how and when to use them. Brushing up on your basic first aid, or better yet, taking a Wilderness First Responder[1] course, can pay dividends when a small or intense medical emergency arises on the run. From blisters to cuts, dehydration, sprained ankles to broken limbs, there is possibility of injury and being prepared to deal with the variety of situations is critical. The very minimal kit I carry includes an ACE wrap, emergency bivy, ibuprofen, BodyGlide™, Band-Aids and triple-antibiotic ointment. Having extra clothing to keep warm, extra calories, lights and batteries for a slower evacuation are additional considerations.

Watch

The timepiece that you wear around your wrist can be a simple timer or as evolved as pinpointing your location. The question is how much information do you want? With functionalities like GPS, route tracker, mileage, lap splits, altitude, distance, heart rate and temperature, there is plenty of information you can log about your run. Each of these help you build awareness in your training and give you perspectives to compare in your training log. Technology desires are specific to each runner and it requires research to ensure you find the model that meets your needs.

Music

When Apple™ released the first iPod Shuffle, I finally succumbed to the aid of music. Before, I refused to carry the extra weight of a mini-disc or cassette player, but with the small Shuffle device and my ensuing summer of the Grand Slam, the $100 investment made a lot of sense. Since then, countless devices have evolved to transport your music while running.

I find there are times that an upbeat tune helps quicken my pace and other moments when I want to completely absorb the quiet of my surroundings. If music is your choice, I encourage you to be aware of your surroundings and fellow runners. You should always be alert to potential danger, whether vehicles, humans or animals. While racing you need to be able to hear alerts from other runners wanting to pass, or communications from volunteers along the course. Wearing only one ear bud and keeping your volume low are good practices. Like trekking poles, some races do not allow the use of headphones.

> Gear: Keep it simple. Make sure it is functional. Update as needed to keep you running.

---

[1] http://wildernessmedicine.com/wfr

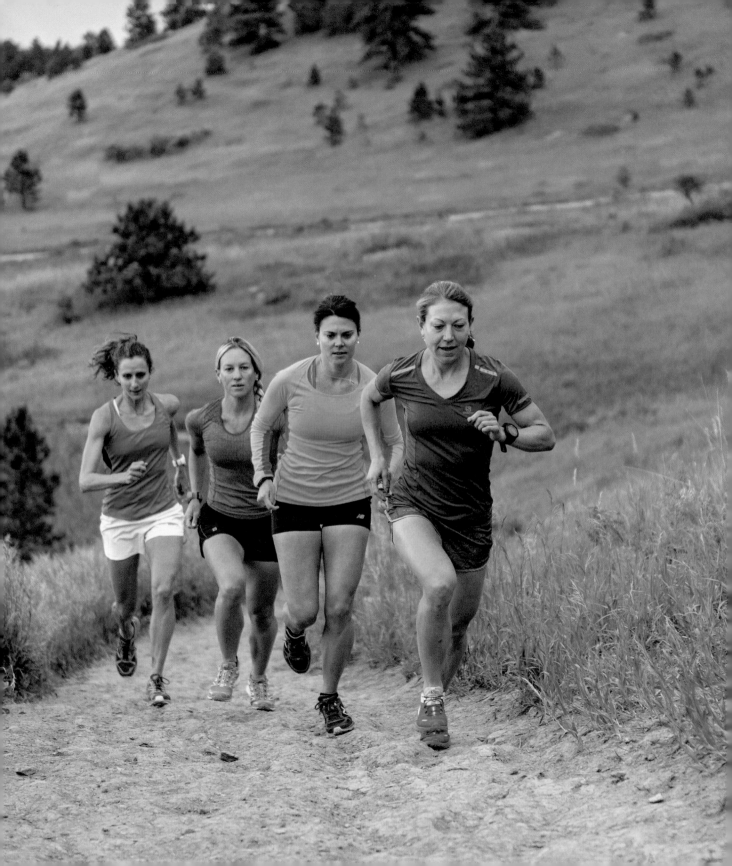

CHAPTER NINE

RUN LIKE A GIRL

(I Encourage Guys to Read This Chapter Too!)

- -

My early days of trail running are synonymous with heckling, stinky sweat and shoes that smelled like aging cheese. Boys. The Scotts (Scott Jurek and Scott McCoubrey) dragged me into the sport and local men filled the Seattle Running Company van every Sunday morning for the Cougar mountain trail run. It was part of the experience at the time; I really didn't know any different. Keeping up made me stronger and faster. Following along I learned nutrition dos and don'ts, to lose all modesty, important foot placement for speedy descents and power hiking to efficiently climb hills.

My trail brothers took care of me. They taught me the important pieces and let me figure out others on my own. They pushed me to try harder and challenged my comfort zone frequently. I learned about the mountains, weather and trail conditions and I am a more capable runner having grown up trail running with the guys. Being let in and taught by the boys showed me how to travel safely and learn a different, more masculine way to cope and process life's challenges. Running with the boys allowed me to work through life's issues pounding out miles.

> "There are not many issues in life a long run cannot solve. Sometimes the run has to be a bit longer." –my quote

Fitting in made me emotionally tough and taught me about interesting gender dynamics. This especially became evident when another woman joined the group; I often felt an adjustment both in myself and in the group dynamic.

- -

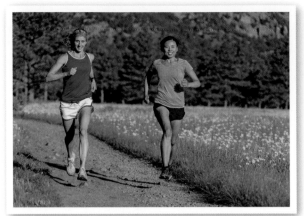
Trail buddies Jenny Jurek and Krissy cruise a few sunny Colorado miles.

As the gender majority shifts, so do the conversations and general feel. The discussion topics change and women's vulnerability and openness set a different tone. We tend to encourage more and taunt each other less, and the camaraderie feels like a warm embrace. We know we have each other's backs physically (I typically put out a hand if someone starts to slide) and emotionally while covering large miles on the trail as we relate and share similar perspectives. All of this creates a different kind of bond.

Moving to Boulder, Colorado and engaging with the running community was the point that my group majority shifted the most significantly; I ran more regularly with women. The commitment to the love of running is the same. The desire to push each other through longer runs is about time in the mountains and catching up on life. When emotions arise we talk about them, rather than pound them out. My advice? As you find your training partners, explore different dynamics and combinations of personalities. The variety will fulfill you in different ways.

Over the years, I have observed growth and change in our sport. One change that I love is watching more women engage. As more strong female role models make their presence in the sport, women see their own strength and capability and feel the desire for this challenge. Because of this, the sport's gender discrepancy is (slowly) coming into balance.

Female athletes, in this case trail and ultrarunners, have a few things to think about as they step into the sport.

WOMEN'S GEAR

Always a creature of function over fashion, learning from the guys did not do my wardrobe any favors. Previously, running clothes, hydration packs and shoes were smaller versions of men's, colored differently. "Shrink it and pink it.[1]" As more women enter the sport the desire to show feminine flare rises, and brands are improving and tailoring products to the female form. Claim your feminine side and dress the part. The products fit better and are designed for our bodies.

In **clothing**, skirts are not only more feminine they tend to function better for our thighs. Reducing the amount of fabric between our legs, as with bulky shorts cut for men, minimizes friction. Wearing tighter fitting, spandex shorts underneath provides a barrier preventing skin-on-skin rubbing and chafing. Similarly for shirts, a more feminine cut fits better around our arms and chests reducing underarm rubbing and accommodating our frame. Closer fitting products for both men and women feel more streamlined and efficient especially as weather becomes a factor. Bulking clothes, even technical fabrics, will hold more moisture if there is excess fabric.

Next to clothing, **hydration packs** are probably the products that have had to shift the most to accommodate women. As distances increase and we need to carry extra calories and liquids, our need for functional, body specific equipment increases. **Waist packs:** Our narrow waist relative to hips is the exact opposite in our male counterparts. Their square frame (equal waist and hips or, reversed of women, larger waist to hip ratio) typically holds a waist pack in place. On women the pack's tendency is to ride

---

1 Brian Metzler at the Trail Ascent Conference October 2014

up closer to our ribs. Elastic and adjustability in the waist pack will form to your figure and reduce excess movement. Backpack styles make carrying extra supplies more comfortable especially when the fit feels more a part of your person. The vest works the best for me as I can easily access supplies from the front pockets and I do not have to remove my pack too often. The key for the feminine form is having adjustability through a couple of well-placed straps to dial in the pack for your frame. Play with opening the chest and tightening the sides (my preference) or cinch the front closed and expand the sides. Try different pocket configurations and definitely fill the pack with your gear to experience what is too much and where to best access your supplies.

A few thoughts on **footwear** are mostly focused on the last of the shoe. This applies for both men and women: it is important to have a shoe that fits your foot and assists your biomechanics (Gear, Shoes, page 181 and Tricks of the Trade, Shoes, page 18). With the boom of running came a market for footwear and there are many brands that make many models. You will find something that fits you. Specific to women, our feet tend to have less volume, so it is important to find a shoe that doesn't bunch or feel bulky. Our biomechanics are also different, mainly because of the angle from our hips to our knees. Core and strength work will support proper biomechanics and running in a well-fitted shoe can help prevent injury. There are more tips on footwear in the gear section, but I wanted to address these two points for women when buying shoes.

Utilizing accommodating design lines and different materials allows brands to fit the female figure so that we can revel in the experience with products made specifically for us. Male or female, you want your gear to fit you.

WOMEN RACING

To this day, the relative fewer number of women in the sport has created a rare luxury. At ultramarathon races, the bathroom lines favor women. But in all seriousness, lining up at an ultra during my early competitive years often meant toeing the line with a lot of testosterone. Starting out of the gates I had to hold my own and jockey for position along the trail with bigger, more muscular frames. I appreciate that they saw me as their equal and didn't pussyfoot around gender formalities, and fortunately, trail runners are generally a kind folk that encourage each other and step aside for a faster paced competitor. You don't see people elbowing or pushing others to the ground. In fact, you're more likely see a competitor stop to pick someone up after falling on a slippery section.

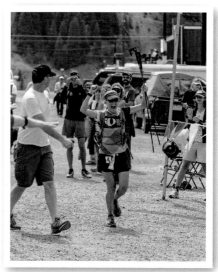

Race Director Dale Garland greets Darcy Piceu as she spots the rock in her first Hardrock 100 win. 2012.

As the finish line nears, and our desire to surge home increases, I found it not uncommon to contest for position with the other gender. Many times as I have approached a male competitor later in a race and asked to slip by I've been met with a surge in their pace. Just as many times I continued at my pace, only to catch up once again and ask the same question. Depending on his endurance and level of ego that is preventing him from letting me by, this process will continue until he is depleted. Eventually, his pace subsides and I scoot by wishing him well. It's called getting chick'ed, and as women's endurance ability grows, men understand that it is not about gender, it is about training. My advice is to run your race, no matter your gender. Do not get caught up in someone else's surges to prevent you passing. Settle in to what is comfortable for you, and what you have trained for and the rest will come.

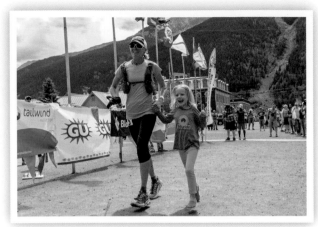

Sophia Piceu Africa adds ease to the end of her Mom's hard effort.

Your race pace comes from your training pace and motivation to speed up can be found in training partners. It is a good idea to have a variety of training paces available to you. You do not always want to feel pushed to your max. Likewise, you will need that sustained quicker turnover on your tougher workouts so that you improve your baseline. A good way to find well-matched running partners is to join a group run and settle in to a pace that feels good for you. Look around and see who you are keeping pace with, who is just ahead and even behind. Your training buds are within sight!

Pregnancy

I can only speak to this from observation and conversations with my fellow female ultrarunning mommas. I am continuously in awe of the female body's ability to create another human being, and the mothers who continue to run through pregnancy and the newborn years take this to another level for me. I do not recommend training for or running an ultra while pregnant, but I see the importance of maintaining fitness.

Every body is different, every pregnancy and birth is unique. The level of fitness that you bring to the pregnancy is an important consideration. Work with an obstetrician who understands your current fitness and your running mind. Together create the safest and most realistic pregnancy fitness plan. Letting your body experience the pregnancy should be foremost. It will tell you what it needs, what is comfortable and what is prohibited. Morning sickness, cramps, pressure on your bladder and other organs will all factor in to how much physical activity you are able to manage. Maintaining fitness will help your mind and movement will help with pregnancy symptoms. Moderating your activity and, again, listening to your body, is what will help you enjoy your pregnancy training and not overdo it.
Some tips include:

➔ Exercise at a conversational pace or wear a heart rate monitor. Most doctors recommend keeping your heart rate below 150—this of course depends on your level of fitness.

➔ Pay close attention to your hydration and recovery.

➔ Wear supportive clothing as your belly size increases. Ex: Wear a belly band while running. A simple band around the base of the belly will help with the bouncing.

➔ Communicate your fitness desires with your doctor to create the best plan.

Menstrual Cycle

Everyone, men and women alike, will deal with highs and lows related to their training and life challenges. However, it seems to me that elevated and changing levels of hormones on a monthly basis is an experience specific to the female body.

I feel it is important to maintain your period. Bleeding on a regular cycle is typically a sign of health and a happily functioning body.[1] Amenorrhea,[2] loss of menstrual cycle, has the potential to create numerous problems for our long-term health, most notably osteopenia or osteoporosis. Women who diet or who

1 Birth control methods, including IUOs, will alter a monthly cycle while still being healthy.
2 Amenorrhea. (n.d.). Retrieved March 30, 2015 from Wikipedia: http://en.wikipedia.org/wiki/Amenorrho

exercise at a high level and do not take in enough calories to expend on their exercise will struggle to maintain their normal menstrual cycles. (Reworded from Wikipedia page.) Maintaining proper nutrition, always and specifically while training, is the best way I have found to maintain my monthly cycle. Acupuncture and supplements are additional methods to engage as needed.

Observing my body I can see shifts and changes in my menstrual cycle relative to my fitness. The more fit I am, the less severe premenstrual symptoms are. Cramping, heavier periods and moodiness are more prominent during the offseason. During ovulation, I typically feel more tired, no matter my training. I have found that consistently supplementing my nutrition with Floradix,[1] an iron and herb supplement, helps maintain my energy levels. It is important to check in with your healthcare provider to ensure proper supplementation for your body's needs. Note that these needs will change with pregnancy, as you age and your training increases/decreases and there are potential health risks with excessive iron intake.[2]

It is helpful to take note of your cycle and how you feel during the various stages. If you pay attention, you will notice a difference in your food cravings, your energy level and how your body responds to training. By making notes in your calendar you can learn how to manage your body and deal effectively with your period through training and racing. I've found that when I sleep more, hydrate extra and eat more clean foods (like vegetables, protein and whole grains) in spite of my cravings for cheese and chocolate, my PMS symptoms (cramping, fatigue and foggy brain) are more manageable. Maintaining my training in spite of PMS symptoms also helps lessen their impact. Ideally timing your races to avoid your period makes for one less race day factor. But unfortunately, this tends to be out of our hands.

Running with Boys:

Cigars. That is what we called them. I added to the crewing entertainment with the most feminine and foreign thing to my five-person, all male crew. My second 100 mile race in less than three weeks and my period started 10 hours before Dale Garland, the Hardrock 100 race director told the field of 125 lucky runners to "Get outta here!" Some races start with a gunshot, others with a blow horn. The Hardrock 100 kicks off at 6 a.m. with a hearty yell of encouragement from the RD followed by hoots and hollers from the bleary-eyed morning crowd. And my crew of guys added a box of tampons to the crew kit knowing that they would have to hand me one each time we met.

No matter your gender, sharing trail time to chat, train, push each other and support each other is an amazing experience, especially when shared with a close friend. The more miles we run, the more raw and more exposed we become. All costumes and filters are stripped away and our communication is real. We are vulnerable, and we show our true selves. It is often said that a friend made on the trail is a friend for life.

1   Iron. (n.d.). Retrieved March 29, 2015 from Flora Health: http://www.florahealth.com/product_az_usa.cfm?sbyletter=F&prod_id=205
2   National Institutes of Health: Office of Dietary Supplements. (2015). *Iron: Dietary Supplement Fact Sheet*. Retrieved from: http://ods.od.nih.gov/factsheets/Iron-HealthProfessional/#disc

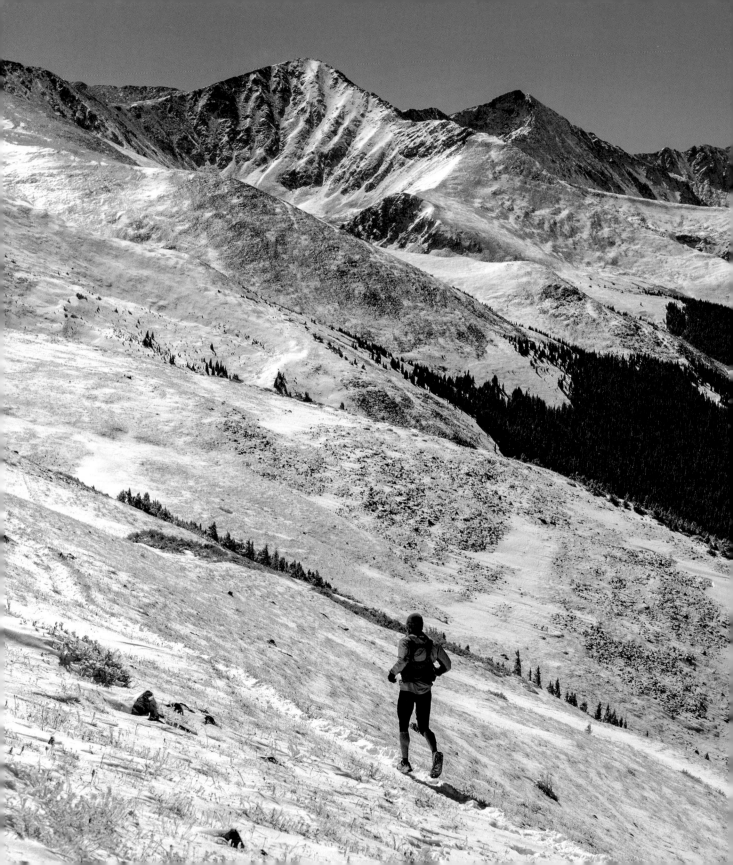

CHAPTER TEN

DIG DEEP AND DISCOVER

"You are better than you think you are, and you will do more than you think you can." —Ken Glober, *founder and former Leadville 100 race director.*

Ultrarunning has the ability to show us who we are at our core, and as Ken Glober notes, this can often mean discovery of a better, more capable person than previously perceived. You will have breakthroughs in your training where you catch glimmers of your potential. When challenged on race day, your ability to move through a rough patch to accomplish your goal may surprise you. The choices you make and the behaviors you exude when you are at your most raw, amped or vulnerable state is the true window into the core of your being. This is why you are here. Be open to this self-discovery and peer in to see what you are truly made of.

> My first ultramarathon race experience reigns as the best life lesson I have learned through participation in this sport. My worried mother's insistence that I remain alert and "with it" each time she crewed me, or she would make me stop, ensured I projected my best demeanor at every aid station. Finding my smile while I endured my biggest life challenge to that point showed me the best approach to any tough life situation. That is to smile.

How you move through these challenges teaches you a lot about yourself and impacts the people around you. If you are grumpy and angry, your demeanor will negatively affect those around you as well as your ability to make the most of the situation. If you can smile and make others laugh, you will move through with grace and everyone will reflect more positively on the experience. Even when you are hands-on-knees puking, I truly believe that a smile will help you rebound faster than a pity party. The energy that you project while running has the opportunity to enhance the experience of your training partners, crew, fellow racers and pacers.

Come race day, remember that challenging your mind, body and spirit is part of the goal. You paid for this. Smile, this is fun! Training takes months to be able to stand on the start line, to wander through the mountains and to test your body in extreme weather. You might slip through unscathed, bouncing to the finish holding hands with your crew. Or you might blow up, hit the wall and experience more rough patches than a pair of old jeans. Either way (or something in between), it is part of the learning process to gain insight by observing how you move through situations.

Nearing the 22-mile mark, the sideways rain soaked every square inch of my body. My fingers were wrinkled from saturation and my face was numb from the stinging drops driving into my cheeks. I pushed my hands on my knees to gain the top of the last climb called little Chinscraper and realized that every step here forward would be the farthest I'd ever run. The fourth aid station was in sight and Ma stood at the front with her hood cinched tightly around her face. She waved her hands so I could see her and as I got closer, I saw her eyes peer into my soul, double-checking to see if I was with it. Tired and worn down by the weather, I hoped she didn't see too deep to the rawness that was quickly being exposed. I looked straight into her eyes, flashed her a smile as if the sun was shining and birds were chirping. She started to question how I felt and I gave her a hug and swapped my two empty bottles for a single pre-filled one. "I'm good Mama!" I waved over my shoulder with another smile as Uli pulled me out of the aid station determined to keep me on course record pace. As soon as I was out of earshot, my smile-covered rawness surfaced and tears, masked by rain, pooled and poured down my cheeks. Still smiling, I could taste the salty tears on the corners of my mouth. In between the pounding of my feet on the sustained dirt road descent I exclaimed, "This is it! I am so lucky. My Mom is the best. This is the best experience. I'm doing it!" Uli in his pragmatic German tone responded simply, "You have less than two hours to run nine miles."

There will be moments when you think forward progress is impossible. You will have to dig deep and tune in to know when to push and when to pass. Only you can go through the challenge to come out the other side. And it is only when you are on the other side that you gain even more insight to who you are and the perspective of what you are now capable. What was once viewed impossible becomes possible.

When I returned to Chuckanut the following year to crew my then boyfriend, I was remembered as the smiling girl. "You smiled every time we saw you!" was a common quote from the kind volunteers. Not only did smiling for Ma keep me in the race, it kept me positive and it influenced volunteers enough to comment a year later.

Darcy Piceut and Krissy running to a new womens Wonderland Trail FKT in 2013. ➜

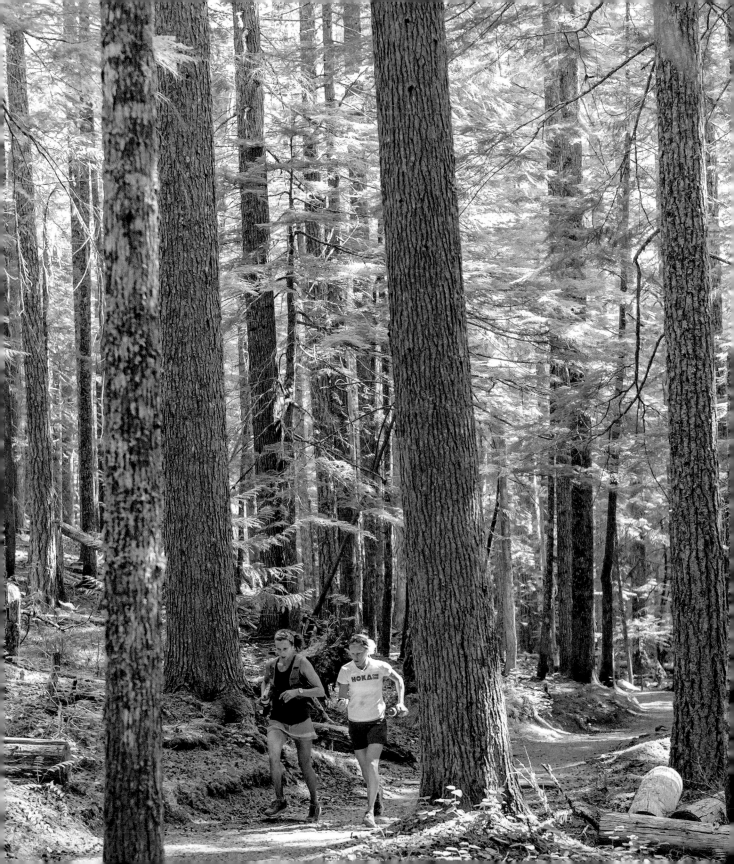

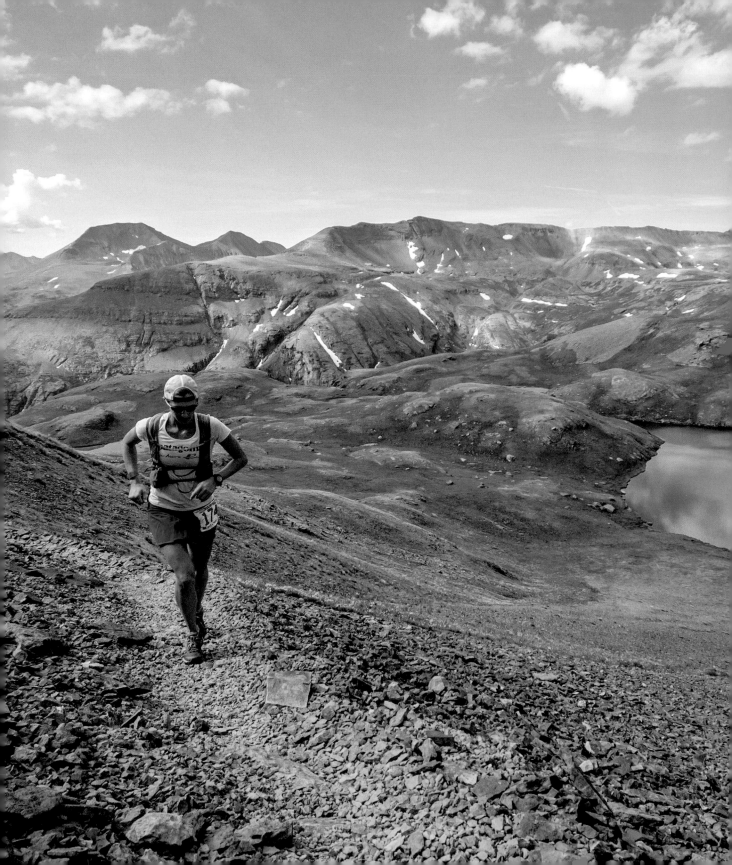

CHAPTER ELEVEN

RACE DAY PREPARATIONS: READY? SET?

- → *Goal Setting (page 199)*
- → *Physical Preparation (page 201)*
- → *Mental Preparation (page 201)*
- → *Preparation, Trail Manners, Race Etiquette (page 202)*
- → *What If's (page 203)*

Through your training plan you have endured miles, experiences, tests of your will and tests of your gear. All of these pieces have built your foundation to help you succeed on race day. It might feel a bit surreal that your big running goal is around the corner, but believe me, you are ready! As you undertake your final preparations, the following will help fine-tune race day.

GOAL SETTING

The first time you set out to run your longest distance, I encourage the finish to be your top priority, whatever it takes. While in practice I have strayed from this guideline because I got caught up in the moment, I know through experience its importance. If you have never run 50 miles before, when you toe that start line **your first goal should be to finish**. Your focus is on the experience and having complete awareness. What do you have to do to keep moving forward? Your body needs to learn what it takes to finish 50 miles or 100 miles before it can take on goal times or placement in the field of runners.

What do you want to achieve in your first ultra run?

_____

_____

_____

_____

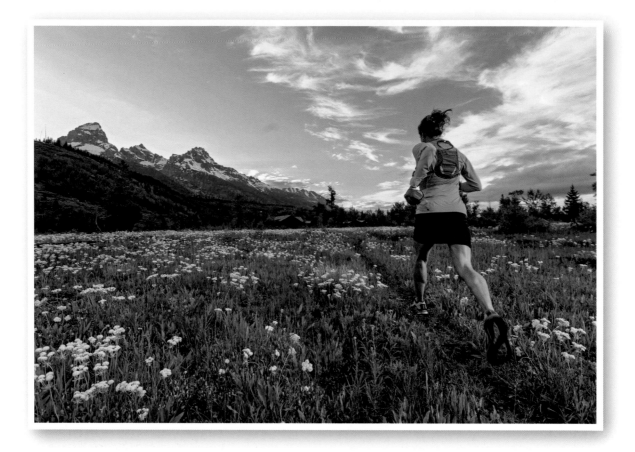

In June of 2011, one week after the finish of my 12th 100-mile race, I had the fortunate opportunity to give a TEDxOverlake Talk.[1] I shared the stories of relearning the following important ultrarunning lessons.

→ Smile. If you are thriving in your experience (taking care of your hydration, nutrition, pacing–run your own race) then it is likely that you will.

→ Make sure those around you are enjoying their involvement in your run. Sharing the experience is a gift. Make it wonderful, special and unique.

→ Use these first two goals to carry you through the first half to two-thirds of your race. Then, and only when 1 and 2 are achieved can you turn on the competitive drive. Now it is time to work toward any icing on the cake goals, those beyond finishing, including placement.

As you visualize your race (guidance below) allow yourself the space to dream about your best effort. That may include a finish time or placement among the field. This is your A race. An A race is when everything is going better than planned. My first Wasatch 100, the stars aligned. Having these goals noted, and secondary to finishing, are motivation to accomplish lessons 1 and 2. When you arrive to the point that you know you will finish, then you can let these dreams kick in and power you to your finish.

---

1 Online link: http://youtu.be/Y7QaqazOv_A

It will be helpful to write out your goals and share them with your crew.

→ Finish: List realistic times and aid station procedures that will ensure this happens.

→ Better than expected: You are moving along well, most everything is seamless and your splits are encouraging a solid finish time. Have splits for this potential and a plan with your crew for how to execute the final miles.

→ The stars align: You are floating over the trails, your fueling is impeccable and pushing for a goal time and/or placement is within reach. The excitement will be hard to control; work with your crew to maintain efficiency.

→ The wheels fall off: The day may not unfold in your favor. How will you manage the challenges? Play out the possible scenario with your crew once or twice, but do not dwell on this prior to the race. Just make the just-in-case plan.

PHYSICAL PREPARATION

You trained and prepared for 24–48 weeks, depending on your plan. Breaking it down into manageable sections finds you here, with enough time for a good taper, ready to apply the many lessons learned over the course of your training.

The first lesson, in the very first week of training, was to think about the program in sections. 24–48 weeks is a lot to swallow at once. So is an ultra. As you prepare for your race, think about how you broke down the training, how it built week over week and now you find yourself near the end of that goal.

Similar thinking will apply to your race. While you have visualized different sections of the course and studied the course map and profile, I encourage you to put that overall view to the periphery of your mind. Focus on the first section, the time splits you've prepared for your crew and the details of the first aid station. Click off one section at a time. Think aid station to aid station, or break it down to each climb and each descent. You might try landmark to landmark. However your strategy develops, evolve and adjust it as you move through the race.

Along the way, the race is going to throw many challenges at you: weather, aid station supplies, gear malfunctions, crew mishaps (I've been through all of these). You have to be flexible when these speed bumps arise. Recall your training, specifically those long runs that challenged your will and that made you question if you could. You made it through those grueling efforts; you can make it through each section and challenge of this ultra race.

"You run the first half with your body and the second half with your mind."–exact author unknown, uttered by many an ultrarunner.

MENTAL PREPARATION

Visualization and race mentality (both covered in Train your Brain, page 33) are your golden tickets in finishing your first ultra. The key is to anticipate possible challenges of the day and mentally prepare how you want to move through them. During the visualizations, acknowledge the miles that are piled up in your legs and notice the fatigue. Now focus your mind, how do you want to approach those feelings? What will you do? Take another gel? Breathe into it? Smile at someone? Ask your pacer for a joke? Plan ahead for how you will approach and deal with that tough space.

Keep in mind that trials from everyday life (not necessarily related to your running) have huge potential to show up on race day and ultra—especially when you are going your farthest distance to date. You will be raw and vulnerable and therefore susceptible to the impact of all emotions. Awareness is extremely helpful in preempting and minimizing the influences of the possible lows on your race experience.

Also visualize the sense of flow, or the zone, of gracefully floating over the trail with minimal effort; whatever you want to call that perfect form and feeling of effortless running. Visualize yourself moving through the miles with ease. What does that feel like? How will you harness that energy to help carry you farther? How will you share it to encourage the experience of those around you? You should prepare to enjoy the highs as much as you endure the lows.

Finally, as you mentally prepare you need to consider your race plan. Going through the What If section at the end of this chapter will help you think ahead about possible race day scenarios and how you want to handle them.

PREPARATION, TRAIL MANNERS, RACE ETIQUETTE

→ Consistently sleep 8–10 hours per night for at least two weeks prior to your race. The extra rest will reset your mental psyche and let the training set into your body so that this 100 miler is fun! Recharge and get psyched! Store up sleep in that bank account to draw on come race day. (Tricks of the Trade, Sleep Deprivation Training, page 30.)

→ Plan out your gear, but do not overthink it. Get everything dialed a week early so that you are not stressed as the race approaches. (Race Packing List, page 226)

→ Drop Bags—see Crew Support page 178.

→ As you get closer to the race, hopefully you will feel a little nervous, but able to control the nerves so that you don't waste energy on taper tantrums. Instead store the building energy for race day.[1] Read Train your Brain, page 38, question #4.

→ Review your predicted time splits and stick to your goals. Do not get caught up in everyone else's race. Run YOUR race.

→ If the start line quickly narrows to a single-track trail, line up appropriately so you do not hold others up or get stuck in the conga line.

→ If you are on an out and back course, move aside for faster runners and make room on the trail to dance around slower runners. Use your voice to alert runners and other trail users that you would like to pass. Make sure they are stable before passing. Cheer on everyone as you pass and thank trail users for stopping their progress to let you by.

→ Will you race with your music? How will it impact your experience? If so, create an awesome playlist that will motivate you when you need it and keep you steady. Consider wearing only one ear bud so that you remain aware of your environment and fellow racers.

→ Move through aid stations quickly and efficiently. Do not sit. Minimize shoe and clothing changes unless absolutely necessary. Have doubles or triples of your gear so you can swap packs and/or bottles with your crew rather than having to refill. Thank all crew members and volunteers as you depart.

→ Appreciatively acknowledge everyone's participation in your effort as frequently as possible.

→ Stay humble. Respect the distance.

→ Learn confidence. Believe in your training.

---

1 For more positive reinforcement on the benefits of training read: Ransone, J. Ph.D. *Peaking the Endurance Runner for Optimal Performance.* http://www.coacheseducation.com/theory/jack_ransone_oct_01.htm

WHAT IF'S

Before you go into your race you need to realize that even the best race plans will have some hiccups. It is a good idea to have the "what if's" answered for yourself and for your crew. Giving these questions some thought will help minimize the gravity of a race-day situation. There is still the chance that an unplanned scenario will surprise you. In that case, having a general approach on how to handle the highs and lows of the day will get you through.

What if I arrive to the aid stations earlier than my predicted splits?

→ Am I having a good day? If yes, proceed and alert the crew to adjust their time sheet.

→ Did I go out too fast? Take a moment with your crew to reset and settle in to a pace that is manageable. Be aware that having spread a bit too much energy early (Spreading the Peanut Butter, page 35) there may be repercussions later.

What if I arrive later than my time splits?

→ Will I still make the cutoffs? Do I feel I can speed up later? Am I being too conservative?

What if I haven't seen a trail marker?

→ Stop and look around. Do not leave the trail you are on. Wait to see (not very long) if another runner comes along and ask them when they last saw a trail marker. Retrace your steps until you find a marker.

What if I get lost, off course?

→ Mark the trail you are on with your initials (draw in the dirt), this gives you a starting reference point in case you start doing circles. As you retrace your steps to find the course make sure you are watching your surroundings. Note landmarks and view points. Take in the landscape and utilize ridgelines, the sun, water features or other prominent landmarks to guide you in one direction. Take inventory of your supplies. Ask fellow trail users for directions using the name of the park or trail system you are using so they can help guide you in the right direction. Do not wander in crazy directions. It is best to stay put and be found than to wander too far. Remember to continue to manage your hydration and nutrition the best you can. Keeping these up will help you make better decisions.

What if the weather goes south?

→ Protect your body warmth. Dress in your extra clothing before you are cold. Get out of the wind and rain if possible when you stop to add layers. Keep fueling. It is easy to be distracted by bad weather or to be frustrated by the excess clothing (gloves, mittens) that makes it difficult to eat. Fuel is important to keep you moving which will generate warmth and allow you to finish.

What if I run out of water or fuel miles from the aid station?

➜ First, do not stress.

➜ Possible solutions: Ask a fellow runner for a sip or a gel if they have extra. Keep your eyes open for clean water sources along the trail. Think positively about the situation and manage your energy output so that you can arrive at the next aid station.

➜ Take time to rehydrate/refuel at the next aid station by drinking little bits when you arrive, while you prepare your gear and as you leave. Consider taking an extra water bottle and a few extra calories over what you originally planned. Sip and eat a little more frequently, rather than gulping large quantities all at once.

What if I blow up? DNF Plan?

➜ How will I handle the blow up? (See Train your Brain, question #5 page 40)

➜ If I determine I cannot run anymore will I walk it in? Will I finish no matter what? (Barring any medical issues.) It is important to think about your finish. Are you there to race (goal time and/or place) and if you are not achieving your goals will still you finish? Are you there to finish no matter what, even if that means walking in the last 30 miles? (I have done this.) Knowing the answers to these questions before you start will help you in the tough moment of decision.

What if I don't achieve my goal?

➜ Your goal in your first ultra should be to finish. Period. Placement or time goals are icing on the cake.

➜ If you don't finish, write about your experience soon after race weekend. Pay attention to how not finishing makes you feel—this will be fuel to your fire later. Sufficiently grieve the DNF, but do not focus on it as failure. See it as a learning experience on how you will excel in your next race. (See more Chapter Five, Train your Brain, Question #7.)

CHAPTER TWELVE

GO!

(This should be read the night before, and re-read race morning before starting)

- -

Breathe. This is your day. It is time to enjoy everything you have put in to your body and mind since you picked up this book and commited to your goal.

Review your time sheet and lock in your splits as segment goals to get you through the day. Run YOUR race.

Remember, this is fun! All you have to do today is eat, drink, run and enjoy.

Work with your crew to have the best race and ensure everyone enjoys the experience.

Be flexible and roll with the day while sticking to your intentions.

Be grateful to everyone, especially yourself.

Smile.

Notes for race day:

_____

_____

_____

_____

_____

_____

_____

_____

- -

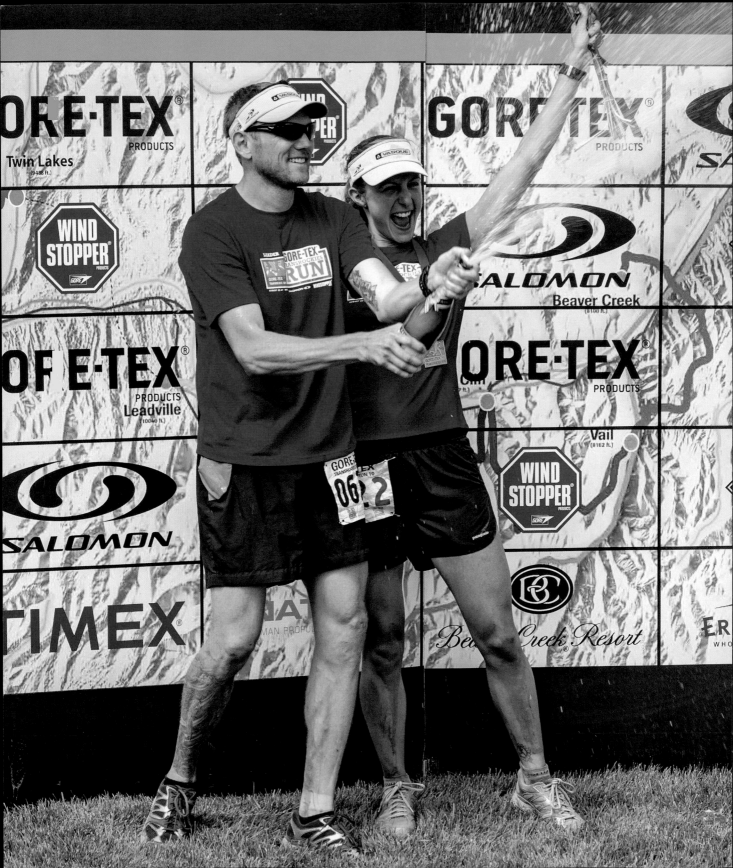

CHAPTER THIRTEEN

RECOVER

- -

Recovery after an ultra event is every bit as important as running the race. I will not leave you to deal with this on your own. Before you start planning the next run, let's make sure you are ready.

Immediately following the run, Celebrate! So many steps, highs and lows have brought you to this point. You finished! Celebrate! Show your gratitude to those that helped make it possible. Acknowledge all that it took to reach that finish line. Laugh. Smile. Cry. Whatever it takes to feel your accomplishment.

Then, slip into your recovery mode. You have trained your system for months to receive proper nutrition in your recovery windows. Post race is no time to slack on taking care of you. Hydrate consistently with your favorite beverages. A few celebratory beers are fair game, just be sure to match each with plenty of water. Shower, sponge bath or at least change into dry clothes. Removing the crusty clothes and layer of sweat, sunscreen, trail dust and whatever else may have attached to you is a helpful piece in starting the recovery process.

Do not be surprised by increased swelling in your legs and hands and even overall puffiness in your body. You have just run the farthest distance (likely to cause some tissue damage) of your life and edema (swelling) is your body's natural response to injury or inflammation. Get your feet up, hydrate, wear compression (if that has worked for you) and try to rest/sleep. Your legs may be jumpy and endorphins pumping may make it challenging to get comfortable at first. As your body heals and recovers you will process the excess fluid.

The most common question after you finish your race will be, "so, what is next?" It is easy to jump back in to training, set the next race goal and charge ahead. Your mind might even fool yourself into thinking you are ready for another long race. The other option is to play the more conservative card.

My go-to response for the "what is next" question is, "to celebrate!" Be in this moment. Reflect on all of the preparations, the race and now the accomplishment of a huge, long-term goal. Celebrating the accomplishment is part of the experience. Not celebrating is like forgetting to put candles on a beautiful baked and iced cake. You trained, cake. You raced, icing. Top it off! Ice cream, candles, the whole bit. Even if you did not finish the race, take this opportunity to reflect and appreciate the many steps it took to come to this point. There will be a finish that you get to celebrate in the future. For now, acknowledge all of your work, the many experiences and the journey.

← Bryan Dayton starts the celebration of our 2010 Transrockies Team win.

- -

As you bask in the accomplishment (for as long as necessary), check in with your body. Are there any aches, pains or tweaks that came up during the race that are sticking around? Do you need to tend to blistered feet? Chafed thighs? Black toenails? Then move to your muscles. Through the months of training leading up to your race you have taught your body to recover. Your muscle soreness may be intense, or it may disappear quickly. This will depend on your nutrition and hydration during and after the race as well as your recovery response. Will an ice bath help? Should you schedule a massage? Try some light movement to see how everything feels. (See Post Race Week Recovery schedule, page 232 for some options.)

Long after your muscle soreness disappears, there is a deeper level of recovery that needs time. This necessary time is relative to the distance you ran; the longer the race, the more recovery time is needed. Do not be surprised if fatigue and increased appetite continue after your muscle soreness dissipates. Your body is communicating its needs. Listen. I believe that there is an impact to your immune, endocrine, and nervous systems that is difficult to measure and fully understand. I have told coaching clients and friends on multiple occasions to give at least two weeks after a 100-mile race to fully feel the effects. In the first week, your endorphins are high and if you had a great race, you might feel invincible. Please wait. If you still feel this way two weeks later, then perhaps you are recovering well. It is my experience in observing myself and many others that the second week after the race is when everything settles. Exhaustion sets in, appetite rages and mental clarity suffers a bit. These responses are normal; you just spent all you had saved up in that bank account. You need to build those reserves again with time, rest and good nutrition.

While depleted, a possible emotional response could arise. You may be more sensitive or have a shorter fuse than normal until you find your balance again. Be aware of any edginess and be careful making emotion-driven decisions during your recovery.

How long before you run again? This depends on your recovery response time, your desire and your schedule. I recommend taking at least 10 days to two weeks (especially after a 100-mile race) before making any significant training decisions. (It took me three months to recover from the Hardrock 100 in 2007.) Allow your body to go through the settling period and maintain recovery awareness beyond muscle soreness. When you start to feel balanced, rested and back to a "normal" appetite then consider increasing your training. During this down time, I definitely encourage movement and active recovery. Flushing the body and maintaining running form (as long as you are not injured) are both helpful to recovery and to keep the mind positive and engaged in the whole process.

WHAT IS NEXT?

- -

➜ *Next Race (below)*

➜ *Race Specific Improvements (page 210)*

➜ *Personal Growth (page 211)*

The possibilities are endless in the world of ultrarunning. On a personal level, you can challenge yourself to run a faster time or a further distance, or to improve your experience through better training and preparation. Thumbing through magazines, sharing stories at finish lines and clicking through countless race websites will open your mind to additional challenges and racing opportunities. The primary piece that I would love to see is the integration of the ultrarunner mindset into your daily life.

NEXT RACE

Now that you have finished an ultra, you get to decide where this sport will take you. Was that a once-in-a-lifetime, check off the bucket list experience? Or are you hungry for more? With this accomplishment under your belt (buckle if you ran a 100-miler!) you might dream of bigger mountains or faster turnover. Your goals might include travel and experiencing trails unlike those you regularly run. For example, if you live in the plains but desire a course profile that mimics a heart attack, you will have to be creative with your training.

➜ Your speed workouts (because the flat plains do not include varying elevation) will be your biggest benefactors as they increase the mitochondrial density (the greater the density, the faster and longer athletes can train/run).[1] This also applies to people with busy schedules. Intensity gives you the best return for your training time. Remember, you should not run every workout at a high intensity; you always need recovery in between.

➜ Including eccentric lifting, mainly with your quads, with your core strength exercises to help strengthen your muscles in preparation for the downhill beating.

➜ Travel to train. Seek out training adventures on terrain that mimics your course. Schedule a long back-to-back training weekend around a trip to a bucket list adventure run. (Ex: Wonderland Trail around Mount Rainier in three days, Zion Traverse, sections of the John Muir Trail.) Training in different landscapes will give you valuable physical experiences and train your brain for confidence when you are out of your normal environment.

Make a conscious choice about your continued involvement in the sport, continue to learn from your experiences and appreciate the exploration, both in the world and in yourself.

---

1 *Trail Runner Magazine*. Issue 102. March 2015. PG. 54. Article "Achieving the Mission Impossible."

A coaching client of mine did the following exercises in preparation for the Chuckanut 50k and was surprised with his minimal soreness. Exercises: squats with weights. Instead of pushing the weight up, slowly lower the weight down. Wall sits. Lunges with weights, again focus on lowering as opposed to lifting.

Race Specific Improvements

After your first ultra, there is opportunity to reevaluate your goals, learn from your experience and push for something a little more. Refer to your training plans and review the notes you made to yourself.

How can I improve my training? Where should I take more recovery? From which workouts did I benefit the most? The least? Can I include more core strength exercise sessions?

_____

_____

_____

_____

What did I learn about my running from my first ultra race? What will I repeat? What will I change? Be specific. Did you devour potatoes or did a certain gel flavor save the day? Clothing? Gear? Crew?

_____

_____

_____

What are realistic training goals for my next ultra? Where can I improve efficiency in my preparation? What should I eliminate?

_____

_____

_____

How can I modify my performance on race day to achieve a faster time? Finish a tougher course?

_____

_____

_____

Personal Growth

Growing up in the sport of ultrarunning has shaped me as a person. The lessons gained from time on the trails, in training and racing, add guidance to my life. Running is my constant; it is there for me daily as a teacher. It helps me cope and process life. Running humbles me through understanding myself better and raises my awareness to my surroundings.

As you journeyed through this training and racing, did you gain insight? Did lessons in self and world awareness bop you upside the head? Did you see your physical limit and move past it? Did you learn a precious lesson in the process?

_____

_____

_____

How can you apply the lessons learned through your training and in your race experience to your life? Absorbing the ultrarunner mindset that helps you achieve seemingly impossible goals and translating it to your daily experience brings your participation in the sport full circle. _This integration moves you from doing an ultrarun to being an ultrarunner. Welcome!_

_____

_____

_____

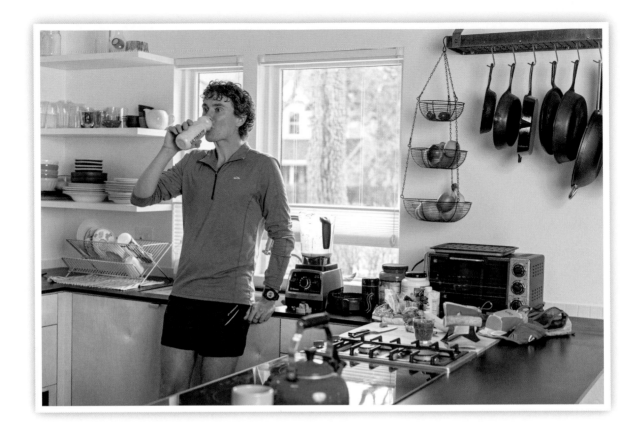

EXTRA PIECES:

Athlete Log Sample

The example below shows one of my training days as an example of how to fill in the training log.

MONTH: _____		
EXAMPLE WEEK	**DESCRIPTION**	**MONDAY**
DATES	WRITE IN SHORT DESCRIPTIONS OF YOUR WORKOUT(S). KEY NOTES THAT WILL HELP YOU REMEMBER THE ROUTE, HOW YOU FELT AND TIME SPLITS ARE ALL HELPFUL WHEN REFERENCING LATER.	AM RUN SANITAS, POORMAN, BETASSO PM SWIM
ELEVATION GAIN	IF YOU HAVE A WATCH THAT WILL TELL YOU ALTITUDE GAIN AND LOSS, IT IS HELPFUL TO UNDERSTAND WHY 5 MILES MIGHT TAKE 2 HOURS VS 50 MINUTES	2800
ELEVATION LOSS		2800
RUN TIME		3:15:00
RUN MILES		18.00
CALORIES BURNED	IF YOU HAVE A WAY OF TRACKING THIS, IT CAN BE HELPFUL TO KNOW WHAT IS NECESSARY FOR YOUR RECOVERY NUTRITION.	
SLEEP	IF YOU NOTE EVEN A GUESSTIMATE OF YOUR SLEEP YOU CAN GAUGE WHY A WORKOUT FELT GOOD OR BAD, OR IF YOU ARE MORE TIRED THAN NORMAL AT THE END OF THE WEEK.	8:00:00
RESTING HEART RATE	BEST TO TRACK YOUR RESTING HR FIRST THING IN THE MORNING BEFORE YOU GET OUT OF BED. TRACK THIS CONSISTENTLY AND YOU CAN TELL WHEN YOU ARE CONSISTENT AND HEALTHY, OVERTRAINED OR GETTING SICK BY CHANGES IN YOUR AVERAGE. THE EASIEST WAY TO MEASURE IS TO COUNT YOUR PULSE FOR 20 SECONDS AND MULTIPLY BY 3.	47
CORE/STRENGTH TIME		
BIKE TIME	THESE ARE ALL NUMBERS, EITHER TIME OR MILEAGE THAT WILL TOTAL AT THE END OF THE WEEK.	
BIKE DISTANCE		
YOGA TIME		
EXTRA...	A CELL TO TRACK ANY OTHER WORKOUTS YOU INCORPORATE.	0:40:00
ATHLETE NOTES	INCLUDE ANY NOTES THAT YOU WERE UNABLE TO FIT IN THE WORKOUT DESCRIPTION CELL. I LIKE TO INCLUDE THOUGHTS ON HOW I FELT DURING THE WORKOUT, OR HOW I RECOVERED HERE.	PM SWIM WAS MELLOW, A NICE COUNTER TO THE HARD MORNING RUN & A GOOD FLUSH TO THE BODY

Athlete Log

I believe the more you write down about your training, the more you will understand what systems work for you. Customize your log so that it is something you will fill in daily; if there is too much information you will not take the time. I've included a blank spreadsheet with multiple data points as a place to start.

MONTH: _____

EXAMPLE WEEK	MONDAY	TUESDAY	WEDNESDAY	THURSDAY	FRIDAY	SATURDAY	SUNDAY	WEEKLY MILEAGE GOAL
DATES								
ELEVATION GAIN								
ELEVATION LOSS								
RUN TIME								
RUN MILES								
CALORIES BURNED								
SLEEP								
RESTING HEART RATE								
CORE/STRENGTH TIME								
BIKE TIME								
BIKE DISTANCE								
YOGA TIME								
EXTRA...								
ATHLETE NOTES								

Core Workout Ideas

COMBO 1

First core strength exercise workout of the week
Knee Hugs. One-legged squats. Lunges. Long jump burpees. Bicep curls. Tricep dips. Crabbie Patties. Crunches. Bridge leg lifts.

Second core strength workout of the week
Curtsey lunges. Deadlift. Golfer swing. Donkey kicks. Stabilizers. Bicep curls. Tricep dips.

COMBO 2

First core strength exercise workout of the week
Long jump burpees. Lunges. Calf raises. Toe raises. Jane Fondas (both). Push-ups. Bridge leg lifts. Kettle bell swings.

Second core strength workout of the week
Knee hugs. Quad stretch. Long jump burpee. Warrior 3 with dumbell. Donkey kicks. Stabilizers.

COMBO 3

First core strength exercises workout of the week
Knee hugs. One-legged bicep curl to shoulder press. Warrior 3 with dumbell. Doggie hydrant. Tricep push-ups, jump! Crunches.

Second core strength sorkout of the week
Kettle bell swings. Body weight squats. Deadlift. Push-ups to row. Jane Fondas. Crabbie Patties.

Core Strength Exercise Descriptions

* You may find YouTube videos to help demonstrate these and other helpful core strength exercises.

➔ **EXERCISE**
Knee hugs (warm up).

Description
Stand tall. Pull one knee up to your chest, hold for a second, then release back to standing. Alternate legs.

Instructions
Do 10 reps on each leg to warm up the hips and hamstrings.

Great For
Loosening up tight hips and hamstrings. Warming up before workout.

➔ **EXERCISE**
One-legged squats.

Description
Balance on one foot, hold other foot just off the floor to your side or in front of you. Holding your arms extended at shoulder height or higher, helps with balance. Squat on your standing leg to about 45–60 degrees (do not go to 90 degrees), push your butt back and keep your knee over your ankle. Keep your foot flat on the floor and your hips aligned (do not let one hip dip lower than the other). As you return to standing, concentrate on contracting your inner quad muscle.

Instructions
Do 15 to 20 reps each leg. Build up to multiple sets. To make this even more challenging and to engage more of your stabilizing muscles, you can stand on a half Bosu ball or other wobbly surface.

Great For
Stabilizing pelvis, strengthen the gluteus medius. Strengthening inner quads.

→ EXERCISE
Calf raises.

Description
Stand on a low bench or the bottom stair with the balls of your feet on the edge of the stair and your heels over the edge. It is good to have a handrail or wall near for balance. Raise up on your toes to flex the calf, then back to level. You can drop your heels a little below level on each rep to gain more extension. Variations: 1) Turn your toes inward, heels out (pigeon-toed) for a set. 2) Rotate your toes outward, heels touching for a set.

Instructions
Three sets of 15–20. Or one set of each of the three variations.

Great For
Calf strength.

→ EXERCISE
Toe raises.

Description
Stand on a low bench or the bottom stair with the heels of your feet on the stair and your toes over the edge. It is good to have a handrail or wall near for balance. Raise your toes to flex the shin, then lower the toes back to level. You can drop your toes a little below level on each rep to gain more extension. Variations: 1) Turn your toes inward, heels out (pigeon-toed) for a set. 2) Rotate your toes outward, heels touching, for a set.

Instructions
Three sets of 10–15. Or one set of each of the three variations.

Great For
Keep shins strong and hopefully prevent shin splints.

→ EXERCISE
Jane-Fonda's bent knee.

Description
Lay on your side and curl your legs to roughly 90 degrees, bending at the waist and knees so that your body is kind of like an "S" but with sharper angles. Tighten your core, keep your feet together and lift the top knee and foot to almost parallel to the floor. From parallel, rotate from your knee to raise your lower leg, ankle now higher than knee. Engage your glutes through the motions. Return to your start position reversing the movements. Do sets on each side.

Instructions
Do equal counts on each side. You might start with 15–20 reps on each side. As you build up you can do two–three sets.

Great For
Our glutes need constant attention to keep them engaged. Runners are notorious for not engaging glutes when running. Keeping them strong will help. You also need to focus on engaging glutes while running.

→ EXERCISE
Jane-Fonda's straight leg.

Description
Lay on one side with legs straight and stacked. Drop top leg behind bottom leg so toe of top leg touches heel of bottom leg. Raise top leg to 45 degrees from hips, then return to position behind lower leg without resting upper leg on the floor. Focus on lifting with the glutes. Do sets on each side. Play with the position of your toe (extend foot, flex foot, point foot towards ground) to vary the exercise.

Instructions
Do equal counts on each side. You might start with 15–20 reps on each side. As you build up, you can do two–three sets.

Great For
Our glutes need constant attention to keep them engaged. Runners are notorious for not engaging glutes when running. Keeping them strong will help.

→ **EXERCISE**

Lunges.

Description

Stand square, feet at shoulder width, knees slightly bent, hands on hips. Step forward with one foot, bend both knees to 90 degrees, your back knee will barely touch the ground. Do not let your front knee bend forward of that ankle, return to standing and switch legs.

Instructions

Start with 10–15 lunges on each leg for one set. Start with two sets. As you gain strength and balance, you can add light hand weights, with arms extended at sides or curl opposite arm/bicep as you lunge.

Great For

Core, quads, hamstrings and flexibility.

→ **EXERCISE**

Curtsey lunges.

Description

Stand square, feet at shoulder width, knees slightly bent, hands on hips. Lunge behind and at an angle behind your standing leg, like when you would curtsey, but over-exaggerate it like in a lunge, bending both knees to 90 degrees. Return to standing and switch legs.

Instructions

Start with 10–15 lunges on each leg for one set. Start with two sets. As you gain strength and balance, you can add light hand weights, with arms hanging along your sides or curl opposite arm/bicep as you lunge.

Great For

Core, lateral quads, glutes and flexibility.

→ **EXERCISE**

Plank, aka stabilizers.

Description

Lay flat on your belly to start. Place your palms under your shoulders, your elbows should point toward the ceiling. Do a push up. Align your shoulders over your palms or shoulders slightly in front. Hold your body flat, balancing on your toes. Hold your belly tight, and think about tucking your pelvis toward the floor to keep your butt in line with your back and not up in the air. Hold position for 30–60 seconds. You can also do this on your forearms. Bend your elbows to 90 degrees and keep your shoulders in line with your elbows.

Instructions

Stabilizers can include a rotation from plank to side plank, back to plank and then to the other side. Hold each position for 30–60 seconds, adding on the advanced movements as you feel stronger. Do two–five rounds.

Great For

Core, shoulders.

→ **EXERCISE**

Side plank, aka stabilizers.

Description

From plank position, rotate to side plank. You can have one palm on the ground with a straight arm, wrist aligned under your shoulder, or position on your forearm, keeping your shoulder over your elbow. Your feet will stack one on the other. Hold for 30–60 seconds. For advanced: Raise your arm over your head, bicep near your ear. More: Lift your top leg and hold. You can also pulse your hips up, try to not let your hips dip below the straight line between your feet and shoulders.

Instructions

Stabilizers can include a rotation from plank to side plank, back to plank and then to the other side. Hold each position for 30–60 seconds, adding on the advanced movements as you feel stronger. Do two–five rounds.

Great For

Core, shoulders.

→ EXERCISE
Crunches.

Description
Lay on your back, knees bent so your feet are flat on the ground. You can cross your arms on your chest or interlace your fingers behind your head. Keep your chin away from your chest; do not pull your head with your hands. Your abs will do the lifting, not your arms. These are small, concentrated movements. Contract your abs and press the small of your back into the ground to lift your shoulders off the ground. There are a lot of variations. 1) Legs up: Lift your legs to 90 degrees, feet are in the air and lower legs are parallel to the ground (bend 90 degrees at hips and knees). Contract abs to lift both shoulders and hips off the ground. 2) Bicycle: From the starting position of the first variation, rotate your core as you lift so that your left elbow meets your right knee. Return to neutral and then rotate the other direction so that your right elbow reaches toward your left knee. 3) Obliques: Rotate your bent knees to one side, twisting at you belly button to stack your knees. Keep your shoulders flat on the ground. Crunch/lift using your side abs (oblique muscles) to lift your shoulders off the ground. 4) Lower ab leg lift: Start laying flat on your back, legs straight. I like to prop my hands under my lower back for stability. Using your lower abs, lift your legs off of the floor. Raise and lower your legs controlling the movement with your abs. 5) Scissor or flutter: From the fourth variation position, maintain legs about 6–12 inches off of the ground. Scissor: Move your legs to cross your feet one over the other, then return to hover position and cross the other direction. Flutter: Flutter kick your legs straight above the ground similar to swimming.

Instructions
Play around with a variety of variations. Do 20–30 reps of each variation. Create a 3–5 minute routine. Focus on the basic position as neutral so that you work your core and do not pull on your neck.

Great For
Abs.

→ EXERCISE
Leg lifts.

Description
Lay on your back, knees bent so your feet are flat on the ground. Lay your arms along your sides. Extend your lower leg (from knee) keeping your knees level. Lower the extended leg to one inch off the ground and lift back to knee height. Repeat for reps. The key piece to this exercise is maintaining your lower back pressed into the floor by contracting your lower abs. You will be able to lift your leg up and down without much effort until you focus on engaging your core.

Instructions
Start with 10 reps on each leg. Build up your number of sets.

Great For
Core.

→ EXERCISE
Leg throw downs.

Description
This is probably my favorite partner exercise. One person lies on the floor. The other stands near their head, typically one foot on either side of their head. The person on the floor grabs the other's ankles for grounding and raises his/her own feet into the air. Keep legs strong and core tight. Press your lower back into the ground through the full range of the exercise. The standing person pushes the horizontal person's feet down. Raise legs back up for more repetitions.

Instructions
The standing person can push the legs to either side, or straight in front. It is a good idea for the standing person to keep a slight bend in their knees for balance as the laying person may pull on their ankles.

Great For
Core.

→ EXERCISE
Crabby Patties.

Description
Remember doing the crab-walk as a kid? Sit on the floor, hands under your shoulders raise up on your feet and hands, belly in the air making a tabletop. Lift left arm and right leg from the floor, balancing on the right arm and left leg. Reach the lifted limbs toward each other in front of you. Try to touch your hand to your ankle. Return to tabletop position and then switch extended limbs.

Instructions
Try to do 10–15 reps on each side. Increase number of sets as you gain strength and balance.

Great For
Core, shoulders, hips and glutes.

→ EXERCISE
Push-ups.

Description
We've all done push-ups! Make sure your back is flat, hips do not sag and core is held tight. Your hands will be a bit wider than shoulder width and your elbows will bend outward from your body, engaging your chest. Variation to help gain strength: Put your knees on the floor while keeping a straight, solid line from knees to shoulders.

Instructions
To build strength, I think it is better to do more sets with fewer repetitions, then to do too many at once. Start with three sets of 5–8 pushups and build up to 10–15 reps per set, then increase the number of sets.

Great For
Chest, upper back, core.

→ EXERCISE
Tricep push-ups.

Description
This is the same idea as above in terms of plank-like body position. The difference is in your arms. Place your hands under your shoulders. As you lower and your elbows bend, keep your arms tight to your body, your elbow should graze your ribcage. This will engage your triceps more than your chest as you push back up.

Instructions
These will be more difficult than regular push-ups for most. Same instructions as above.

Great For
Triceps, core.

→ EXERCISE
Push-up to lateral arm raise.

Description
Keep push-up form. At the top of your push-up, press into your right hand, lift your left hand into the air and rotate your whole body to side plank position with your arm straight up in the air (toward 12 o'clock). It helps to keep a wider stance with your feet and rotating on to the arch of your left foot and outside of your right. Return to push-up position. Do a push-up. At the top of the next push-up switch sides, lifting your right hand into the air.

Instructions
Start with 5–10 reps on each side. Do two–three sets. Hold light dumbbells in each hand to increase difficulty.

Great For
Core and shoulders.

→ EXERCISE
Push-up to row.

Description
Keep push-up form. At the top of your push-up, hold the upper plank position and press into your right hand. Pull your left hand into your chest, your left elbow will laterally be in line with your shoulders. It helps to keep a wider stance with your feet. Return to push-up position. Do a push-up. At the top of the next push-up switch sides, pulling your right hand to your chest.

Instructions
Start with 5–10 reps on each side. Do two–three sets. Hold dumbbells in each hand to increase difficulty.

Great For
Core, shoulders and lats.

→ EXERCISE
Pull-ups.

Description
These are the most difficult core exercise for me, and are arguably the most beneficial. Hang from a solid bar or pull-up board. Cross your ankles and bend your knees. Engage core, back, arms to pull your body up so that your chin reaches bar height. Fully extend back to hanging position.

Instructions
This might be good to do with a friend to hold/support your feet, giving a little boost as needed or with a weight assisted machine until you can use good form to pull up your weight. Do 3 sets of as many reps as you can.

Great For
Back, core and arms.

→ EXERCISE
Long jump burpee.

Description
Stand square, feet shoulder width apart, knees slightly bent. Bend your knees and jump forward with both feet, swing your arms to help. That is the long jump. Then a burpee: drop your hands to the floor just in front of your feet. Jump your legs back to push-up position, do a push-up, jump feet forward toward your hands, stand up. That is one rep.

Instructions
Try to do 10 reps. Increase number of sets as you gain the strength and balance. This will raise your heart rate if done quickly in succession.

Great For
Everything.

→ EXERCISE
Lunge behind, kick.

Description
Stand square, feet shoulder width, hands on hips for balance. Lunge your left leg back behind you, bend both knees to 90 degrees and press back up to standing. As you return to the start position continue with your left leg (balance on the right) and bring it forward to kick, controlled by your core (do not throw your foot in front of you) bring the leg through from your hip, knee bent and then extend your knee to a kick in front of you. Then move back through neutral to step behind into the lunge again on the same side. Repeat for all reps each side.

Instructions
Try to do 10 reps on each side. Increase number of sets as you gain the strength and balance.

Great For
Legs and core.

→ EXERCISE
Deadlift.

Description

Form is key on this Olympic lift. Start with light weights (maybe 5 lbs in each hand). Stand square, feet shoulder width, hands hold weights in front of you, arms extended. Shrug your shoulders, up and back, hold your shoulder blades on your back. With knees slightly bent and back completely flat, core contracted, bend at the hips to lower the weights (with straight arms, shoulder blades locked on to your back) to just below your kneecaps. Return to standing reversing the controlled motion. Use your legs, push into your heels, keep your back flat, arms in front. Shrug shoulders again, up and back to make sure they are still in the right position once you are fully standing. Repeat keeping good form.

Instructions

Start with two-three sets of 10 reps. You can increase reps and weight as you get stronger. Standing sideways to a mirror is a great way to watch your form.

Great For

Hamstring strength and flexibility.

→ EXERCISE
Kettle bell swings.

Description

Hold kettle bell in both hands, arms hanging in front of you. Stand with legs wider than shoulder width, feet flat on the ground pointed slightly outward, knees bent in a squat. Do not bend your knees past your ankles. Be careful with your back. Be sure to keep your core strong, pelvis tucked and back straight. As you stand up from squat, swing kettle bell up to shoulder height using the strength of your legs as they press to stand, your tight core and lastly your arms.

Instructions

Start with a light weight to learn the movement. I recommend two-three sets of 10 reps. You can increase reps and weight as you get stronger.

Great For

Core, shoulders and legs.

→ EXERCISE
One-legged bicep curl to shoulder press.

Description

Stand on one leg with a dumbbell in the same hand of the leg that is off the ground. Slightly bend the standing knee for balance. Bend the raised knee to hip height and hold. Start with the weight at your hip, do a bicep curl with the dumbbell and continue the motion to extend your arm into a shoulder press. Return the weight to your hip in the reverse motion and repeat 8-10 times. Then switch sides.

Instructions

Start with a light weight to learn the movement. I recommend two-three sets of 10 reps. You can increase reps and weight as you get stronger.

Great For

Shoulders and balance.

→ EXERCISE
Warrior 3 with dumbbell.

Description

Stand on one leg with a dumbbell in the same hand of the leg that is slightly off the ground. Slightly bend the standing knee for balance. Hold the weight at your hip. Extend your arm down toward the ground, straight arm, flat back, shoulders square to the ground, shoulder locked (like a deadlift) as you extend your lifted leg straight behind you. Your back and leg should make a "T" to your standing leg, and your arm with the weight should hang straight down from your shoulder. Return to standing and repeat 8-10 times on the same leg. Then switch sides.

Instructions

Start with a light weight to learn the movement. I recommend two-three sets of 10 reps. You can increase reps and weight as you get stronger.

Great For

Hips, balance and stability.

→ EXERCISE
Golfer swing.

Description
Stand tall. Raise your hands to shoulder height (bend elbows so your hands are in front of or just outside of your shoulders) for balance. Raise one leg slightly off the ground. Pretend your leg is the golf club—keep your body in between two panes of glass, one pane on your front and the other on your back. Swing raised leg out laterally toward hip level and return to standing.

Instructions
Fifteen reps each leg. Increase number of sets as you gain strength. You can also add small weights in your hands.

Great For
Hips, balance and stability.

→ EXERCISE
Donkey kicks.

Description
Kneel on hands and knees, 90 degree angles at hips and knees. Engage your core to help stabilize the position. Use your glutes to extend one leg behind you, keep the knee at 90 degrees, bottom of foot parallel to the ceiling. Press your foot up engaging your glutes to make the motion happen. Small controlled movements. Repeat on same leg for 10–15 reps then return to hands and knees to switch.

Instructions
One set is 10-15 reps on each leg. Increase number of sets as you gain strength.

Great For
Glutes.

→ EXERCISE
Doggie hydrant.

Description
Kneel on hands and knees, 90 degree angles at hips and knees. Engage your core to help stabilize the position. Use your glutes/hip to lift one leg out to your side to hip level, keep the lifted knee at 90 degrees. Return to hands and knees. Repeat on same leg for 10–15 reps, then switch.

Instructions
One set is 10–15 reps on each leg. Increase number of sets as you gain strength.

Great For
Glutes.

→ EXERCISE
Tricep push-up, jump!

Description
Use form description for tricep push-up. At the top of the tricep push-up, engage your core to jump your legs up toward your hands. Your feet may land around the side of your hands in a wider stance. Then jump your feet back to tricep push-up position and repeat.

Instructions
Try to do 10 reps. Increase number of sets as you gain the strength.

Great For
Triceps, core.

Crew Packing List

CREWING FOR: _____

- ☐ ID or Passport
- ☐ Boarding Pass

CREW EQUIPMENT

- ☐ Black Diamond Sprinter Headlamp
- ☐ Julbo Sunglasses
- ☐ Sunscreen
- ☐ Chapstick
- ☐ Packable Chair
- ☐ Baby Wipes or Washcloth
- ☐ Knife, Spoon

CREW CLOTHING

- ☐ Patagonia Baggies
- ☐ Patagonia Cordelisse Sport Bra
- ☐ Patagonia Cross Back Tank
- ☐ Patagonia Merino 2 Long-sleeve Light Weight Zip
- ☐ Patagonia Capiline 1 Silkweight T-shirt
- ☐ Patagonia Lightweight Merino Crew Socks
- ☐ Patagonia Better Sweater Beanie
- ☐ Patagonia Truck Hat
- ☐ Patagonia Better Sweater Gloves
- ☐ Waterproof Mittens
- ☐ Patagonia Houdini Jacket
- ☐ Patagonia Torentshell Waterproof Stretch Jacket
- ☐ Vasque Trail Shoes

CREW GEAR

- ☐ Electronics Chargers
- ☐ Coffee Mug
- ☐ Water Bottle
- ☐ Toiletries

- ☐ Towel
- ☐ Camera
- ☐ Pillow
- ☐ Sleeping Bag
- ☐ Sleeping Pad
- ☐ Books and Journal
- ☐ iPad
- ☐ iPod
- ☐ Earbuds or Speaker
- ☐ French Press

NUTRITION

- ☐ Snacks
  - ☐ Trail Butter
  - ☐ Carrots, Apples
  - ☐ Pita Chips
  - ☐ Protein (jerky, baked tofu)

POST-RACE CLOTHING

- ☐ Patagonia Organic Cotton T
- ☐ Patagonia Serenity Pants
- ☐ Patagonia UltraLight Down Hoodie
- ☐ Flip Flops
- ☐ Patagonia Vanilla Beanie

REMINDERS

- ☐ Change voicemail (alert out of office/home)
- ☐ Notify credit cards (international travel)
- ☐ Set up email auto-response

Fuel Chart

Please note that all nutritional facts are based on amount per package. The chart does not reflect serving sizes.

Brand	Product	Calories / package	Carbohy-drates (g)	Sugar (g)	Dietary Fiber (g)	Protein (g)	Fat (g)	Flavor	Sodium (mg)	Potassium (mg)	Calcium (mg)	Magne-sium (mg)	Caffiene (mg)	Chlo (mg)
Bearded Brothers	Bars	283	27	20	4	6	13	Fabulous Ginger Peach	14					
Bob's Oat Bar	Bar	360	54	16	6	6	14	Coconut						
Clif	Bar	260	41	21	4	9	8	Pecan Pie	170	170				
Clif	Bloks	200	48	24		0	0	Strawberry	100	40				
Clif	Builder Bar	270	30	22	3	20	9	Vanilla Almond	220	150				
Clif	Drink	80	20					Cranberry Razz	250	50				
Clif	Luna Protein Bar	170	21	15	3	12	4.5	Lemon Vanilla	160	85				
Clif	Recovery Drink	160	30	28		16	0	Chocolate	15	140				
Clif	Zbars	120	23	12	3	2	3	Chocolate Chip	95	105				
Clif	Luna Bar	190	24	11	3	10	7	Honey Salted Peanut	260	135				
First Endurance	EFS	96						Fruit Punch	300	160	100	150		
First Endurance	Liquid Shot	400	100	50	0	0	0	Vanilla	400	290				
First `Endur-ance	Ultragen	320	60	60		20	0	Fruit Punch	350	200				
GU	Chomps	180	46	22		0	0	Strawberry	100	80				
GU	Recovery Brew	240	46			8	2	Chocolate Smoothie	190	390				
GU	Roctane Electrolyte Caps								140			9		125
GU	Gel	100	20	5		1	1.2	Peanut Butter	65	60				
Hammer Nutrition	Endurol-ytes	2 capsules							80	50	100	50		120
Honey Stinger	Waffles	160	21	14	1	0	7	Honey	55					
Kind	Bar	200	15	5	7	6	16	Caramel Almond Sea Salt	125	200				
nuun	1 tab	7	1					Grape	345	97	13	25		
SaltStick			1 capsule						215	63	22	11		350
Skout	Bar	170	32	21	4	3	4.5	Blueberry Almond	60	200				
Succeed!	S!-Caps	1 capsule							341	21				
Trail Butter	Energy nut butter	800	32	16	12	20	68	Mountain-eer Maple	140					
V-Fuel	Gel	100	23	6		0	1	Mountain Berry	10	15		5	10	
Vega Sport	Recover Bar	260	27	16	3	15	11	Chocolate Peanut Butter	150					
Vega Sport	Sustain Bar	230	27	19	4	4	14	Coconut Almond	10					
	Avocado	234	12	1	10	2.9	21			708				
	Date	20	5	4.5	0.6	0.2	0			47				

Race Budget

Plan ahead for the expenses of your race to reduce financial stress.

	A PRICE PER (DAY)	B # NEEDED	TOTAL = A+B TOTAL
FLIGHT	EX: $300.00	2	$600
ENTRY FEE			
TIME OFF WORK (HOPEFULLY YOU CAN USE VACATION DAYS AND THIS IS NOT A COST TO YOU)			
MILEAGE			
GAS			
FLIGHTS			
RENTAL CAR			
LODGING (HOTEL, HOME STAY, BNB, VRBO)			
MEALS			
BREAKFAST			
LUNCH			
DINNER			
SNACKS			
RUN NUTRITION			
RECOVERY FUEL			
GEAR			
SHOES			
SHORTS			
SHIRTS			
SOCKS			
HYDRATION PACKS			
HEADLAMPS			
TREKKING POLES			
WATCH			
BLISTERSHIELD/BALMS/OINTMENTS			
CREW TOTAL COSTS—DISCUSS WHO WILL COVER THESE COSTS AHEAD OF TIME			
LODGING (HOTEL, HOME STAY, BNB, VRBO)			
MEALS TOTAL			
BREAKFAST			
LUNCH			
DINNER			
SNACKS			
CREW GIFT -THIS DOESN'T HAVE TO COST MONEY, BUT SHOULD BE THOUGHTFUL			
TOTAL			
UNEXPECTED 10% BUFFER	*THIS IS ONLY FOR PLANNING PURPOSES AND IS NOT INCLUDED IN YOUR TOTAL		

Race Packing List

RACE: _____

- ☐ ID or Passport
- ☐ Boarding Pass

RACE EQUIPMENT

- ☐ Ultraspire Isomeric Handheld Bottles
- ☐ Ultraspire Surge Pack
- ☐ Pro-Tec Patella Knee Bands
- ☐ Black Diamond Icon Headlamp
- ☐ Black Diamond Sprinter Headlamp
- ☐ Batteries
- ☐ Julbo Access Sunglasses
- ☐ Black Diamond Ultra-Distance Trekking Poles
- ☐ Sunnto Ambit 3 Watch
- ☐ Sunscreen
- ☐ Newskin
- ☐ Blistershield
- ☐ Butt Balm
- ☐ Chapstick
- ☐ Arnica Gel
- ☐ iPod Shuffle
- ☐ Earbuds
- ☐ Baby Wipes or Washcloth

RACE CLOTHING

- ☐ Patagonia Strider Pro Shorts
- ☐ Patagonia Cordelisse Sport Bra
- ☐ Patagonia Draft Tank
- ☐ Patagonia Merino 2 Long-sleeve Light Weight Zip
- ☐ Patagonia Capiline 1 Silkweight T-shirt
- ☐ Patagonia Lightweight Merino Run Anklet Socks
- ☐ Patagonia Capilene 4 Expedition Weight Beanie
- ☐ Patagonia Duckbill Truck Hat
- ☐ Buff Headband
- ☐ Patagonia Lightweight Merino Glove Liners

- ☐ Waterproof Mittens
- ☐ Patagonia Houdini Jacket
- ☐ Patagonia Houdini Pants
- ☐ Patagonia Torentshell Waterproof Stretch Jacket
- ☐ Patagonia Torentshell Waterproof Pants
- ☐ Vasque Trail Shoes

TRAVEL GEAR

- ☐ Pro-Tec Orb
- ☐ Pro-Tec Stretch Belt
- ☐ Phone Charger
- ☐ Coffee Mug
- ☐ Water Bottle
- ☐ Toiletries
- ☐ Towel
- ☐ Nail Clippers and File
- ☐ Camera
- ☐ Pillow
- ☐ Sleeping Bag
- ☐ Sleeping Pad
- ☐ Books and Journal
- ☐ iPad
- ☐ French Press
- ☐ Power Adaptor, charging cords
- ☐ Ziplock™ Bags—helpful to sort food/gear

NUTRITION

- ☐ Race
  - ☐ Clif Shot Gels
  - ☐ Clif ZBars
  - ☐ Clif Bloks
  - ☐ Gu Brew Electrolytes Caps
  - ☐ First Endurance EFS Liquid Shot
  - ☐ First Endurance Ultragen
  - ☐ Trail Butter
  - ☐ Medjool Dates

- ☐ Travel Snacks
  - ☐ Trail Butter
  - ☐ Carrots, Apples
  - ☐ Pita Chips
  - ☐ Protein (jerky, baked tofu)
  - ☐ Salad
  - ☐ Baked Sweet Potato
- ☐ Supplements
  - ☐ Flora Probiotics
  - ☐ Floradix Pills
  - ☐ First Endurance Optygen
  - ☐ First Endurance Multi-V
  - ☐ Emergen-c
  - ☐ Flora 7-Sources

POST-RACE CLOTHING

- ☐ Patagonia Organic Cotton T
- ☐ Patagonia Serenity Pants
- ☐ Patagonia UltraLightDown Hoodie
- ☐ Flip Flops
- ☐ Patagonia Vanilla Beanie
- ☐ Compression Tights
- ☐ Injinji Compression Socks
- ☐ Patagonia Trucker Hat

REMINDERS

- ☐ Change voicemail (alert out of office/home)
- ☐ Notify credit cards (international travel)
- ☐ Set up email auto-response
- ☐ Crew gifts

Race Time Sheet

This time sheet will allow you to plan your splits and gear necessary for all aid stations and crew spots along the route. I think it is a good idea to plan the entire race (first sheet) and then par down the spreadsheet to the information that is relevant to your crew. Finally, having contact information (assuming you are pulling friends from different walks of life) will allow your crew members to remain in contact before and during your race.

START	AID STATION 1	AID STATION 2/ CREW 1	EX: AID STATION 2/ CREW 1	AID STATION 3	AID STATION 4	AID STATION 5/ CREW 2	AID STATION 6
RACE MILE			29.7				
SEGMENT (miles from previous aid station)			5.9				
SUB-24 HR			11:20 AM				
SUB-30 HR			12:55 PM				
CUT-OFFS			1:50 PM				
PACER			N/A				
HYDRATION			New hydration pack & 1 hand-held. Both filled with ice & water. Handheld with EFS drink.				
NUTRITION			4 Clif Shots, 2 pkgs Bloks, 5 TB filled dates, GU Brew Electrolytes				
ADDITIONAL GEAR			Sunglasses, Visor. Apply sunscreen. Please take headlamp.				

CREW PERSON	EMAIL	PHONE	ARRIVAL	DEPARTURE

Racing to Train. 100-mile prep–weeks 15 and/or 30

Racing to train might leave you feeling a little confused. Because you are training through the 50k (week 15) and 50M or 100k (week 31) you will not be as rested and tapered for the race. You might not have your best performance on race day, but know it is because you are working within your training and this is a part of strengthening and preparing the mind and body to be ready for your bigger goal.

I encourage you to run a 50k around week 15 and a 50 miler around week 30 of your 100-mile training plan, especially if this is your first time training for 100 miles. I realize that the training races you pick may not fall exactly on weeks 15 and/or 30. Use what you have learned about training and the weeks that are laid out in the training plan to finagle the workouts to work with the race date(s) that you are able to utilize in your training. If you are looking for more mileage and experience, and you come to this training with more under your belt (perhaps you already sport a 100-mile finisher's belt buckle) then running a 50-mile race at week 15 is possible and you can look for a 100km race at week 30.

Use these races to test out all of your gear. You will be amazed at how your favorite shirt, which you've run 20 miles in, doesn't work for 50 miles. It may even chafe you. The waist belt that you have been running with might squeeze your belly over this long haul and effect digestion forcing you to look into a different method to carry your fluids and foods. Sunscreen. Skin lubes. Supplements. Sports foods. Real foods. Give all race day necessities that you are thinking about using or consuming on your 100-mile race a try during these training races. When you finish, jot down notes about what worked and what didn't. These will be helpful to review as you pack and plan for your big day.

Pay attention to feelings (physical and emotional) that arise during your training race. It is your goal to figure out how to manage them. Basically, what does it take to keep you moving forward?

➜ Do you need more calories?

➜ Are you hydrated?

➜ Are you too warm?

➜ Too cold?

➜ If it is muscle soreness, or a more intense pain, do you need to stretch? Would a short walk break help?

➜ How is your motivation level?

➜ Are you engaged in the race or wishing you were elsewhere?

➜ How can you make the most of each moment? Push the pace? Or completely pause to take in the view?

➜ What will it take to make it through the next section?

➜ Is there something your crew might be able to do when you arrive? (Massage? Pep talk?)

Be in the moment and figure out how to move through all feelings that arise; this awareness will pay huge dividends for your goal race.

What did you learn from these training races that will help better prepare you for your 100-mile debut?

*Gear Notes:*_____

_____

*Physical notes:*_____

_____

*Mental notes:*_____

_____

Finally, your goal is 100 miles. These mid-training program races are to help you prepare for it. You may or may not have your best run during one of these training races, but do not put much emphasis on either. (Okay—you should celebrate if you set a PR!) Ideally you want these to be learning experiences as you train and prepare for the 100-mile race day.

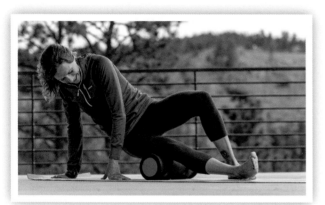

Recovery Movements

Always loosen up with at least 10 minutes of cardio or easy running before stretching. There are many great resources available for stretching practices, methods and theories. Move about and find what works for you.

The following are my top-five favorite stretches. I typically hold each for 5–10 seconds then switch sides and repeat until I feel fluid or for as long as I have time.

→ Side Stretch: Stand tall. Raise hands/arms straight overhead. Grab left wrist with right hand. Stretch up and then over to the right keeping your hips and shoulders facing straight ahead (as if pressed between two panes of glass) gently pulling your left side open. Keep your legs strong. Return to standing and switch your grip to stretch your right side.

→ Quad Stretch: Stand tall, hands/arms at your sides. Bend your left arm at the elbow, palm face up out to your side. Balance on your right foot. Lift your left foot behind you and catch the top of your foot in your left hand. Keep your knees aligned and your pelvis tucked. If you cannot hold your foot in your hand, use a strap or a belt to loop around the top of your foot. Use a running bud or a steady object to balance if you wobble too much. Aim to balance on your own. Switch legs.

→ Hip Stretch: Stand tall. Step your right foot behind in a lunge, balancing on the ball of that foot. Pretend your feet are on railroad tracks about 6–10 inches apart (instead of on a line) so that you can maintain balance. Bend your left knee forward to no more than 90 degrees while keeping your right knee straight. Focus on stretching the front of your right hip. EXTRA: Raise both arms above your head and stretch (like in #1 Side Stretch) to your left to open the hip more. Switch legs to stretch your left hip.

→ Hamstring Stretch: You can do this sitting or standing, legs parallel to each other. Keep a slight bend in your knees and reach for your toes bending at the waist and aiming to keep a flat back. EXTRA: you can spread you legs into a "V" and stretch to the middle and to each leg.

→ Calf Stretch: This is best done on a slant board. Standing with ball of foot on the roughly 45-degree angle, lean forward with a straight leg, you should feel this in the higher portion of your calf and perhaps behind your knee, then back off the stretch. Then bend your knee forward to stretch different muscles. You will feel the stretch move down to the lower part of your calf. Switch legs.

Self Massage

I am a big advocate for self massage for daily maintenance in addition to working with a licensed massage therapist. As I understand, foam rolling and more focused Orb rolling™ (because of the shape of the roller) help increase blood flow and release soft tissue adhesions, also known as myofascial release. Both of these benefits can improve recovery time and help prevent injury. A few key areas I like to focus on with a foam roller or Orb are listed below. As you become more comfortable moving around on these self-treatment tools explore other areas.

Foam Rolling

➜ Hamstrings: This is probably the most common foam rolling position. Sit on the ground with the foam roller under your knees. Prop yourself up on your hands to pick your butt off of the ground and roll forward and backward from your knees to your butt.

➜ Calves: From the same starting position as hamstrings, now roll from your knees to your ankles.

➜ Quads: Press yourself into forearm plank or push-up position. Place the foam roller under your hips. Lower your quads on to the roller and move back and forth from your hips to your knees.

➜ IT Band: A very common tender point on runners that can easily turn into injury. Similar to the quad rolling, start in push-up position and rotate to one side. Place the foam roller at your hip and roll the lateral length of your leg to you knee. It is likely that you will have "speed bumps" (tighter areas) along each side, and possibly more on one leg than the other. Adjust your pressure by lifting or lowering more of your body weight on to the roller. This is probably the most intense foam rolling position. For even more intensity, use the Orb instead of the foam roller.

Orb Rolling™

➜ Hamstring attachment points: A tricky spot on runners is right below our buttocks where the hamstrings insert. Rolling the Orb in this general area, up onto the butt cheek and down along the backside of your leg will help loosen tightness and work to relieve that pulling feeling that builds with the combination higher mileage running and extended periods of sitting.

➜ Back: Standing against a wall, place the Orb between your back and the wall. Roll up and down the wall using your pressure to increase or decrease the intensity.

➜ Calves: Same as above, use the Orb instead of the foam roller for more focused self massage.

➜ IT Band: Same as above, use the Orb instead of the foam roller for more focused self massage.

Post-Race Recovery Week

Congratulations! Are you still celebrating? Do your muscles remind you of your accomplishment as you move?

MONDAY: Rest.

Light stretching and movement will help flush the stiffness you feel in your legs.

TUESDAY: 45 min cardio.

This is more about movement and less about anything cardio. Building up a sweat will feel good and leave you a bit more fluid after. Pay attention to any pains or tweaks that might linger from your race. Ice, massage and treat as necessary to encourage a speedier healing process.

WEDNESDAY: 3 miles steady pace. Core strength exercises.

Take it easy. Walk to start and let your body warm up to the movement. It might be best to run solo so that you do not get caught up in someone else's pace. If getting out the door to test your running legs feels like a huge undertaking, switch today's miles with Thursday's rest. You do not *need* to run yet. This is more of a physical check-in than a run.

Move through some of your favorite body weight core strength exercises. This is more for the flexibility/elongating component and not about building strength.

THURSDAY: Rest.

Hopefully the stiff and sore feelings are leaving your legs. As they dissipate, tune in to your level of fatigue, appetite and other recovering systems. What do you notice as the endorphins wear off?

FRIDAY: 5 miles steady or 35–60 min cardio.

Today and tomorrow's runs are simply to get you moving. The mileage is not mandatory; both days are suggestions. See how you feel. Repeat this week for additional recovery. Take note of where you are able to move more compared to the first post-race recovery week.

SATURDAY: 5–8 miles.

SUNDAY: Rest.

Not including injury, you should see notable improvements at this point. Imagine what another week will bring. Take it easy. Look at your finisher's award, share stories with your crew, write a blog post or note highlights in your journal. Reflect on what that race meant to you now that you are a week out.

ACKNOWLEDGMENTS

Thank you for the opportunity to work with you through your first ultra race experience. Witnessing newbies' curiosity, spark and wide-eyed enthusiasm for ultrarunning renews my spirit and love for our ultrarunning community. Take care of our sport, learn about its early roots and integrate all that you learn into life. I look forward to sharing trail time and hearing your stories.

THANK YOU

→ Ma & Pa and Seester: consistent cheerleaders and the best, unconditional support a daughter/sister could imagine.

→ Christine, Will, Marissa and Meg at Page Street for finding me, hearing me and making this project a reality.

→ My coaching clients for their spark and intrigue.

→ Instrumental to my writing process: Don ensured all i's were dotted and t's were crossed before the writing began. Sherry stepped in as the best (self-proclaimed) research nerd a new author could imagine. Dr. Cooper for opening my eyes to the importance of fueling and adding her expertise in these pages. David's red pen kept me inspired to write better. Jeff provided support while editing and during a few road warrior days. Running trails near my home provided motivation and helped avoid hitting the wall on this ultra writing process.

→ My mentors: Scott Jurek, Scott McCoubrey, Steve Loitz, David Horton, Doug McKeever, the old Montrail guard, and many greats from those early Seattle trail days.

→ Fred's ability to capture the passion of trail running and sharing his art in these pages.

→ I am thankful for so many people I have met through running and sharing time on trails. My inspiring running buds. Faces from all over the world: JU, Monica, Jonna, Jackie, Brenda, Ashley, Missy, Roch, Catherine, Toph, Kim, Kathleen, Fid, Ellen, Justin, Pieper, Bronco, Gavin, Chad, Devon, Nathan, Jon, John S., Cherie, Jenn, Kunlong, Dan, Lizzy, Luke, Bryan, Kay, Simon, Terra, Chris, Serena, Kristie, Walter. Our Wednesday girls run: Darcy, Gina, Cassie, Ashley, Kerrie & Tressa. … And so many salty, dirty, soulful runners, I love all of ya!

→ Friends and family from my non-running world that keep balance and reality present.

→ Patagonia, Vasque, Pro-Tec Athletics, Flora Health, First Endurance, Clif Bar, Julbo, Trail Butter and Ultraspire. Sponsors enable athletes to do more with financial and product support, but the true benefit is knowing that these brands believe in what we do and who we are.

ABOUT THE AUTHOR

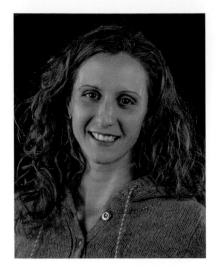

Sculpted, shaped and self-discovered on trails all over the world, Krissy Moehl is thankful for the consistency of trail running in her life. There are so many life lessons to be learned from pushing our limits in natural, beautiful surroundings, that she feels lucky to have found this outlet early in life.

Through her passion for trail running, Krissy has had the opportunity to travel and experience the world. She first discovered the trails after studying abroad in Ecuador, in 1999. She credits the support of her family, the trail running community, her rich life experiences and the open spaces of high alpine terrain for inspiring her to keep moving forward. Through all of life's highs and lows, she has found solace in putting one foot in front of the other.

Despite her relative youth at age 37, Krissy is vulnerable and raw by years of hard miles, and she finds growth, safety and positive influence in the power of wild places. Following her heart through leaving her job, winning on the world stage, negotiating relationships and enduring physically challenging adventures has led to astonishing victories, epic failures and incredible self-discovery.

Krissy appreciates opportunities to explore the world through the lens of running and is thankful for the miles her body continues to let her cover. In addition to running races and traveling, she is an ambassador for Patagonia and Vasque footwear. She race directs the Chuckanut 50k, coaches newbie ultrarunners and enjoys the challenge of public speaking.

Krissy hails from the Pacific Northwest.

TOTALS: 100+ RACES, 55 WINS, 3 FKT'S, 10 EVENTS*

* events are other multi-day, long distance, unscored, ultra fun adventures

- ➜ 100 mile PR 2012 Western States 100 18:29:15
- ➜ 100 km PR 2010 Mad City 100k 8:33:51
- ➜ 50 mile PR 2006 Croom Trails 50 miler 7:12:39
- ➜ 50 km PR 2007 Chicago Lakefront 50k 3:51:48
- ➜ 26 mile PR 2009 Lithia Loop Trail Marathon 3:17:58

Highlights

Date	Event	Time	Place Overall	Female
4/26/13	Ultra Trail Mount Fuji 100-mile race	24:35	25TH	1ST
8/22/13	Wonderland Trail FKT w/ Darcy Africa	22:22	*female supported record run around Mt. Rainier Africa*	
6/23/12	Run Around the Roof of Africa (Kilimanjaro) *270 km, 34,000ft climb*	1ST group ever, only female		
10/20/12-10/27/12	Western States 100 mile	18:29:15	26TH	4TH
9/19/10	Shinetsu Five Mountains 110 km Trail Race *Madarao, Japan*	13:31	14TH	1ST
8/28/09-8/29/09	Ultra Trail du Mont Blanc 166km Trail Run	24:56:01!	11TH	1ST
1/13/07	HURT 100 mile	26:15	2ND tie	1ST
8/19/06	Where's Waldo 100km	11:18	1st overall	1ST
6/25/05-6/26/05	The Grand Slam of Ultrarunning: Western States 100 Mile Endurance Run	20:53:06	36TH	4TH
7/16/05	Vermont 100	18:41	8TH	1ST
8/20/05	Leadville Trail 100	22:03:03	13TH	2ND
9/10/05-9/11/05	Wasatch Front 100 * the youngest and 2nd fastest women to complete the series	26:34*	24TH	3RD
7/13/04-7/14/04	Hardrock 100 mile trail run	29:24:45!	3RD	1ST
9/11/04-9/12/04	Wasatch Front 100 Mile Endurance Run * the youngest and the 5th women in the race's 25-year history to break 24 hours	23:49:47*	7TH	1ST
8/29/03-8/30/03	Tour du Mont Blanc 150 km	29:40	24TH	1ST
3/00	Chuckanut 50k	5:03:41!	15TH	1ST

INDEX